KU-608-495

AIDS & HIV in Perspective

A Guide to Understanding the Virus and its Consequences

BARRY D. SCHOUB

SECOND EDITION

LIVERPOOL
JOHN MOORES UNIVERSITY
AVRIL ROBARTS LRC
TITHEBARN STREET
LIVERPOOL L2 2ER
TEL. 0151 231 4022

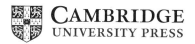

CAMBRIDGE
UNIVERSITY PRESS

PUBLISHED BY THE PRESS SYNDICATE OF THE UNIVERSITY OF CAMBRIDGE
The Pitt Building, Trumpington Street, Cambridge, United Kingdom

CAMBRIDGE UNIVERSITY PRESS
The Edinburgh Building, Cambridge CB2 2RU, UK http://www.cup.cam.ac.uk
40 West 20th Street, New York, NY 10011-4211, USA http://www.cup.org
10 Stamford Road, Oakleigh, Melbourne 3166, Australia

© Barry D Schoub 1999

This book is in copyright. Subject to statutory exception
and to the provisions of relevant collective licensing agreements,
no reproduction of any part may take place without
the written permission of Cambridge University Press.

First published 1994
Reprinted 1995 (twice)
Second edition 1999

Printed in the United Kingdom at the University Press, Cambridge

Typeset in Sabon 10/13pt, in QuarkXPress™ [wv]

A catalogue record for this book is available from the British Library

Library of Congress Cataloguing in Publication data

Schoub, B. D.
AIDS & HIV in perspective : a guide to understanding the virus and
its consequences / Barry D. Schoub. – 2nd ed.
    p.   cm.
Includes bibliographical references and index.
ISBN 0 521 62150 X (hardback). – ISBN 0 521 62766 4 (pbk.)
1. AIDS (Disease)   I. Title.
[DNLM: 1. Acquired Immunodeficiency Syndrome.   2. HIV Infections.
WC 503S376a 1999]
RC607.A26S3738 1999
616.97'92–dc21
DNLM/DLC
for Library of Congress   98-11707 CIP

ISBN 0 521 62150 X hardback
ISBN 0 521 62766 4 paperback

DEDICATION

This book is dedicated to the memory of the hundreds of thousands of fathers, mothers, brothers, sisters, sons and daughters who have perished in this awesome epidemic.

CONTENTS

PREFACE TO THE SECOND EDITION

What has happened to the HIV/AIDS epidemic since the publication of the first edition of this book in early 1994? Globally the epidemic is even worse than anticipated five years ago, although the expansion has been uneven. In the developing world of sub-Saharan Africa it has multiplied threefold and in South and Southeast Asia, sixfold, while in Europe and North America the prevalence of HIV/AIDS has increased only slightly. The science of AIDS has progressed remarkably, providing clinicians with new diagnostic tests to more precisely chart the progress of the disease and assess responses to therapy. In addition, a wide range of new anti-HIV drugs has become available and modern therapeutic regimens are now able to so dampen down viral activity that it is no longer detectable in the blood by highly sensitive diagnostic tests. There are many who now feel that HIV/AIDS has truly become a chronic treatable rather than a progressively fatal disease. These new therapies, however, come with a substantial price tag, putting these hopes well beyond the reach of the great majority of people living with HIV/AIDS. The ethical difficulties that have been such an intrinsic component of HIV/AIDS ever since it was recognized in humankind still persist. In many respects there has been little progress in addressing the fundamental human rights issues surrounding HIV/AIDS and the stark global inequities appear to be widening. Undoubtedly, real progress has been made in the First World – educational programmes have succeeded in modifying risk behaviour and the epidemic curve in these regions of the world is flattening out and people living with HIV/AIDS can look forward, with a cautious optimism, to a considerably longer and more improved quality of life. Protective vaccines are now also on the verge of undergoing clinical evaluation. However, this progress has not, as yet, man-ifested itself in the Third World where the root causes of the disease, poverty and deprivation, are still the engines that drive the epidemic. The most crucial challenge of the HIV/AIDS epidemic still remains – that of being able to provide effective lifestyle alternatives relevant to the devel-oping world, and also to be able to provide effective antiviral drugs and ultimately protective vaccines that are relevant to the financial capacities of the Third World. These challenges will remain as the final test before the claim can be made that HIV/AIDS has been conquered.

February 1998

PREFACE TO THE FIRST EDITION

Since the dawn of mankind, no other disease has so menaced civilization as AIDS. The potential for mass destruction of such large sections of humanity has never been so great as is the case with this disease. In the major cities of the African continent up to one third of the adult population is presently infected with HIV, forming an enormous reservoir of infection which acts as a source for yet further infection of an even greater proportion of men and women, who, in their turn, are now a further source of infection. In no other disease of humans are all those who are infected potentially able to transmit the infection for the duration of their lifetime. Furthermore, most or all of those who are infected will probably also succumb eventually to the disease of AIDS, which will inexorably lead to their deaths within a few years. Over and above this frightful spectre of the disease itself is the stigma and the degradation which is attendant on sufferers from AIDS. Added to all of this is the eagerness of the media, not surprisingly, to sensationalize this disease. It is therefore small wonder that there has been, hitherto, no other disease which has been the subject of such misinformation and misunderstanding and which has led to so much fear, superstition, prejudice and myth, as AIDS.

Many bodies and groups have made, and are making, most commendable attempts at education, with both general and specific programmes targeted at high risk groups. In highly motivated communities such as male homosexual populations in cities such as San Francisco in the USA, the dividends of educational programmes have been gratifyingly visible. However, for the general public, educational programmes often appear to convey mixed messages. On the one hand, the grave risks and the dangers of the transmissibility of HIV by casual sexual contact or sharing of needles are emphasized and highlighted. On the other hand the insignificant risk of being infected by the virus through contacts other than sexual or sharing of needles is equally strongly and reassuringly emphasized. Often, educational messages, however well intentioned, are perceived as being dogmatic and pedantic or trite and facile, or sometimes paternalistic. How often have those of us in the field of AIDS been accused of a 'cover-up', of not telling the true story about AIDS, and of deliberately concealing statistics. No matter how regularly and how forcibly one tries to impress on the man or woman in the street that this virus is not transmitted by breathing in contaminated air or ingesting contaminated food, or touching the sweaty hands of an infected patient, sensationalistic misinformation, sometimes deliberate with mischievous intent to support prejudices and a desire to stigmatize groups, more often than not has greater plausibility with the public.

After a number of years of delivering lectures and seminars to lay, semi-professional and professional audiences, in addition to answering thousands of queries on AIDS and especially with regard to the risks of transmission of the virus, it has become abundantly clear to me that what is urgently needed by the layperson, and often also the professional public, is a text which bridges the gap between scientific literature and educational pamphlets. To distil down and extract from the gigantic volume of scientific literature being generated on AIDS and related subjects in order to create this book has been no easy task. I have had to compromise on the one aspect which I used as a criticism of many current educational programmes, that of being dogmatic. An additional major problem in writing a volume of this nature is the very rapid changes in our knowledge and understanding of the virus and the disease it causes. No other pathogenic organism or disease entity has been so intensively studied and has had such a vast volume of scientific literature published about it. As a result I have had to be, to some extent dogmatic as it would be impossible in a text of this scope to enter into the contrasting views which authorities hold on various aspects of AIDS. However I have studiously avoided being prescriptive as the aim of this book has been purely to provide an understanding of this extraordinary virus, how it produces disease, how the extent of disease is tracked and what steps are being made to control it and why progress in this regard has been so disappointingly slow. Armed with knowledge and understanding, the reader would then be in a better position to evaluate newspaper reports on 'breakthroughs' or accusations of cover-ups, or inflated figures of depopulation of communities and countries and collapse of labour forces and other doomsday predictions. It is my earnest hope that this volume will complement the highly commendable educational programmes of so many dedicated workers while, at the same time, help to put an end to the mischief of the prophets of doom and the bigots.

ACKNOWLEDGEMENTS

This book was written following numerous requests from many different quarters. However it was the encouragement from my wife, Barbara, and also my children, Wendy, Richard and Peter, which provided my main inspiration and motivation and I am deeply grateful for the wonderful support which they gave me. I would also like to record my sincere appreciation to Mrs Vicky Canning of Sandton Literary Agency, South Africa, for her help and encouragement. To my secretary, Mrs Liz Millington, who patiently and with such extraordinary dedication typed the manuscript and maintained such a particularly high level of professionalism and skill, goes my sincere appreciation for contributing so much to making this book happen. Also, to Mrs Marion Taylor, who was responsible for the line drawings, my gratitude for her outstanding contribution and her unfailing willingness to help. I would like to thank my colleagues at the National Institute for Virology, Dr Peter Jupp who was responsible for the photography, and Dr John Sim who assisted with the graphics and also designed Fig. 2.6. Dr David Spencer, head of the Immunodeficiency Clinic of the Johannesburg Hospital, very kindly provided the photographs for Figs. 1.1, 1.2, 1.3, 1.4 and 1.5, and Professor Ron Ballard of the Department of Microbiology, South African Institute for Medical Research, Figs. 4.5, 4.6, 4.7 and 4.8. The electron photomicrographs, Figs. 2.5, 2.7 and 2.8, were supplied by Professor Mike Lecatsas, Professor of Virology, Medunsa University, South Africa. Permission was granted by Mates Healthcare Ltd to use their display card of condoms for Fig. 4.9 and Ileven® for their brochure for Fig. 4.11, the Wellcome Foundation for the picture of zidovudine for Fig. 6.5 and the WHO for permission to adapt Figs. 9.1 and 9.2 from the Weekly Epidemiological Record.

INTRODUCTION

The history of AIDS

The international tracking and monitoring of human disease is one of the major functions of the World Health Organization (WHO) in Geneva. On a national level, disease surveillance and the charting of the origin and development of both infectious and non-infectious diseases is of cardinal importance to the maintenance of public health, and institutions and agencies of varying sizes and formats have been established in most developed and in many developing countries of the world for this purpose. The largest and best known of these institutions is the Centers for Disease Control and Prevention (CDC) in Atlanta, Georgia, USA. The CDC is charged with disease monitoring and surveillance in the USA but also performs the lion's share of international disease monitoring.

Through a very widespread reporting network throughout the country as well as abroad, information and details of human diseases are fed to the CDC. Here it is received by large teams of epidemiologists (scientists trained to investigate the extent and patterns of behaviour of diseases in communities and populations) as well as statisticians and data processors. When required, teams of field workers are sent out from the CDC as well as from more regional health authorities, to obtain more detailed information or to investigate outbreaks or epidemics. On the basis of these epidemiological and as laboratory studies, an ongoing composite of human diseases is maintained. This particularly valuable information is communicated to public health workers and scientists throughout the world by means of regular publications such as the weekly *Morbidity and Mortality Weekly Report*.

It was at the CDC that the first indications of the impending AIDS epidemic became evident in the autumn of 1980. Between October 1980 and May 1981 an alert physician, Dr Michael Gottlieb, together with colleagues at three different hospitals in Los Angeles, became intrigued by a cluster of five young male patients, whose ages ranged from 29 to 36 years, under their care. Two of the patients died and the remaining three were seriously ill. All five men, who had previously been healthy, were diagnosed as having a highly unusual form of pneumonia due to a parasite called *Pneumocystis carinii*. *Pneumocystis carinii* pneumonia (often abbreviated to PCP) had previously been found virtually exclusively in patients with severe suppression of their immune systems caused by drugs or disease. In addition, all of these patients had evidence of having been infected with a virus called cytomegalovirus (CMV) which is similarly common in immunosuppressed patients. All five of these patients were also infected with thrush, which is again characteristic of immunosuppressed individuals. Indeed, in three of the five who were tested there was evidence of marked disturbances in the functional capacities of their immune systems. A further feature of the five men was that all were sexually active homosexuals. None of them knew each other, however, and there did not appear to be a common sexual contact. At this stage this all pointed to an association with a homosexual lifestyle and a sexually transmitted disease.

The first report of these observations appeared in a relatively small unobtrusive insert in the *Morbidity and Mortality Weekly Report* of the CDC on 5 June 1981 (Fig. 0.1). A month later, the 3 July issue carried a similar report of 26 homosexual men, 20 from New York and six from California, with a very uncommon tumour called Kaposi's sarcoma (named after the nineteenth-century Hungarian dermatologist, Moritz Kaposi who first described this skin tumour). Kaposi's sarcoma (often abbreviated to KS) had previously only been observed in elderly men, often of Mediterranean and Jewish extraction, and also in tropical Africa mainly in children and young adults. It was also becoming increasingly evident in patients undergoing kidney transplantation who were on immunosuppressive drug therapy where the tumour was considerably more rapid growing and took a decidedly more malignant course, as was also the case with the 26 homosexual patients now described.

The observation of 26 patients with KS over a 30-month period of time was certainly noteworthy. The New York University Cancer Registry had only recorded three KS cases in men under the age of 50 between 1961 and 1972 at New York University Hospital, and none between 1970 and 1979 at Bellevue Hospital, New York. As with the original five PCP

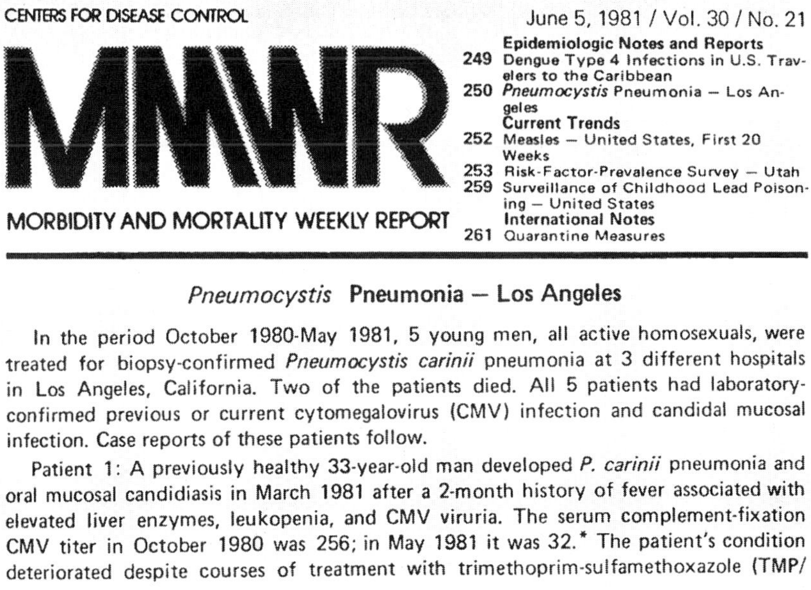

CENTERS FOR DISEASE CONTROL

June 5, 1981 / Vol. 30 / No. 21

MMWR

MORBIDITY AND MORTALITY WEEKLY REPORT

Pneumocystis Pneumonia — Los Angeles

In the period October 1980-May 1981, 5 young men, all active homosexuals, were treated for biopsy-confirmed *Pneumocystis carinii* pneumonia at 3 different hospitals in Los Angeles, California. Two of the patients died. All 5 patients had laboratory-confirmed previous or current cytomegalovirus (CMV) infection and candidal mucosal infection. Case reports of these patients follow.

Patient 1: A previously healthy 33-year-old man developed *P. carinii* pneumonia and oral mucosal candidiasis in March 1981 after a 2-month history of fever associated with elevated liver enzymes, leukopenia, and CMV viruria. The serum complement-fixation CMV titer in October 1980 was 256; in May 1981 it was 32.* The patient's condition deteriorated despite courses of treatment with trimethoprim-sulfamethoxazole (TMP/

Fig. 0.1 Report in the *Morbidity and Mortality Weekly Report* of 5 June 1981 on *Pneumocystis* pneumonia in five male homosexual subjects – the first intimation of the impending AIDS pandemic

patients, the KS patients also had evidence of infections such as CMV, thrush and PCP. Meanwhile a further ten PCP cases in homosexual men were reported from California.

Thus it was at the beginning of the 1980s that the relatively unremarkable few cases of homosexual male patients with unusual infections and tumours heralded in an epidemic of one of the most devastating of all diseases of humankind and one which would have, perhaps, the most profound effect on the practice of medicine of any single disease. Because the disease was obviously transmissible from person to person and because of its striking effect on the suppression of the immune system of patients, it was named the acquired immunodeficiency syndrome, or AIDS.

In 1982 a set of clinical criteria was established which could be used to define AIDS. Armed with this case definition health workers, both in the USA and elsewhere, were then able to set about quantitating the extent of the disease, and monitoring and charting its progress. By May of 1985, in the USA 10 000 cases of AIDS had been reported. Most of them had died within two years of the diagnosis being made. Similarly, in the UK, a national AIDS surveillance programme was established in 1982 by the

Public Health Laboratory Service Communicable Disease Surveillance Centre in London. In that year only three cases of AIDS were reported in the UK. In 1983 there were 28, in 1984, 77 and in 1985, 165. Similar patterns emerged elsewhere in other countries in the developed world, where surveillance programmes were established and the disease looked for. In most cases it was fatal within two years of diagnosis, and it was mostly found in homosexual men and also, to some extent, in persons who injected themselves intravenously with illicit drugs.

Early in 1983 similar vigilance and alertness resulted in a finding of almost equal importance to the original uncovering of the AIDS epidemic. Doctors in Belgium and France became aware that African patients with AIDS appeared to lack the two lifestyle risk factors of male homosexuality and intravenous drug abuse, so characteristic of the disease in Western countries. It also differed with respect to being found equally amongst females as well as males, unlike the marked male dominance (owing to its prevalence in homosexual men) of Western countries. Also, unlike Western countries, the disease appeared to spread mainly by heterosexual contact and was particularly common in female prostitutes. The trail of investigation then led to their countries of origin in Africa and, in the beginning, particularly Rwanda and Zaire, where a vast reservoir of the disease existed and provided a sizeable source of AIDS patients found in Europe, especially in countries such as Belgium.

The discovery of the causal agent of AIDS

From its very beginnings the most striking feature of the AIDS epidemic in the USA and in Western countries was its dominance in the male homosexual population. It was therefore logical to search for clues for the cause of the disease amongst practices or characteristics of this lifestyle. One of the most favoured of the early theories related to the use of so-called recreational drugs, particularly amyl nitrite. This chemical is commonly used by heart patients to relieve angina due to coronary artery constriction, as it is a potent dilator and relaxant of blood vessels. The same effect of amyl nitrite was being utilized by homosexual men to dilate the blood vessels of the penis to prolong erection and heighten sexual excitement. Amyl nitrite also, however, happens to be a relatively strong suppressor of the immune system and its habitual and frequent usage was therefore thought to progressively destroy the immune system and eventually result in the disease of AIDS.

Another of the early possibilities under consideration as a cause of AIDS was semen, which had been known for some time to have immuno-suppressive properties. The link with homosexuality was postulated to be the practice of rectal intercourse. The single-celled mucosal lining of the rectum is far thinner and more friable than the multicell- layered vaginal mucosa (see Figs. 4.2–4.4). Rectal mucosal damage is therefore common in a passive partner in homosexual intercourse, which could well allow the introduction of semen, with its immunosuppressive properties, directly into the bloodstream. Furthermore, detailed studies of homosexuals established that individuals who regularly or exclusively acted as passive partners in intercourse were at considerably greater risk of AIDS than those who were regularly or exclusively active partners. However, an important deficiency in these early theories was that they failed to address the obvious trans-missible or infectious nature of the disease. A number of infectious agents were then postulated as possible causes of AIDS, either acting on their own or in concert with the effects of recreational drugs or the introduction of semen in the bloodstream with traumatic sexual intercourse.

One of the first candidate infectious organisms put forward was a virus that commonly infects humans and is itself known to produce a fairly strong suppressive effect on the immune system–cytomegalovirus (CMV). CMV, so-called because it causes cells that it infects to become patholog-ically enlarged, had been known to be an important cause of disease in humans, especially for its role in congenital infections (infections of the developing foetus) as well as diseases in immunosuppressed individuals. Virtually all patients with AIDS have evidence of infection with CMV and many suffer from the diseases that the virus characteristically produces in immunosuppressed patients, such as pneumonia, which is frequently fatal, infections of the retina of the eye, which may lead to blindness, infections of the bowel, as well as other organs of the body. In addition, one of the important routes of transmission of CMV is venereally. The major problem with the CMV theory is that infection with the virus is itself so common in humans. In most individuals who are infected it is present in a latent or hidden form, as is characteristic of all members of the herpes virus fam-ily to which CMV belongs, and it only produces disease when activated – that is, when some triggering factor causes it to come out of its latent stage and start multiplying to produce an acute infection and then disease. One of the most important triggering factors is suppression of the immune system which usually keeps a vigilant watch over the virus and maintains it in its latent state. Evidence of infection with CMV is found in virtually all homosexual men, irrespective of whether they have AIDS or not, as well as in a large proportion of healthy persons. On closer scrutiny, it soon became apparent that active CMV infection and CMV-related disease, when it was part of the AIDS clinical picture, was more likely to be a secondary result of immunosuppression than a primary cause of AIDS.

A second early contender for the role of the causative agent of AIDS was a virus of considerable veterinary importance but one which hitherto had not been known to cause disease in Man. This virus, the African swine fever virus (commonly abbreviated to ASFV), as the name implies chiefly infects pigs and, as would be consistent with AIDS, it involves the immune system of the animal. The suggestion that the virus may be implicated in AIDS arose from observations by workers at Harvard University that the onset of the epidemic in Haiti, which had at an early stage been thought to be a high risk area for AIDS, coincided with the introduction of the virus into that country. Although in pigs the virus is spread mainly by the bites of infected ticks it has also been shown to spread via semen and blood. Intriguing though the idea was, considerable scepticism greeted the ASFV proposal right from its onset. Compounded with this was the considerable difficulty in testing human specimens for evidence of infection because of the very stringent regulations preventing work with the virus except under very strict containment facilities present only in a few laboratories in the world, as ASFV is such a serious threat to the agricultural industry. Nevertheless, testing that was carried out on material from AIDS patients failed to reveal consistent evidence of infection and the ASFV theory soon disappeared. Other infectious agents, or combinations of agents, were also put forward as possible causes of AIDS, including hepatitis B virus.

Two important scientific discoveries published a decade previously paved the way for the development of a technology that would ultimately enable the causative virus of AIDS to be isolated. In 1970 two biochemists, David Baltimore of the Massachusetts Institute of Technology and Howard Temin of the University of Wisconsin, described and characterized an enzyme whose proposed activities were initially regarded as being biologically heretical. This enzyme, called reverse transcriptase, was responsible for the formation of a deoxyribonucleic acid (DNA) copy from a ribonucleic acid (RNA) template, the reverse order of the accepted sequence in biology (Fig. 0.2). The dogma up to then had been that the genetic material of life forms, which resided in the DNA molecule, directed the formation of its specific and characteristic proteins via a messenger RNA molecule. Thus, the genetic master code, written into the DNA, acts as a template for the intermediary messenger RNA to be manufactured and this RNA, in turn, then directs the cells' factories to make the requisite specific proteins needed by

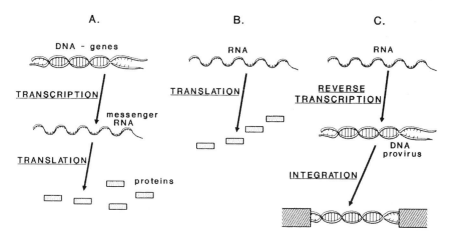

Fig 0.2 The three main types of viral replications: (A) DNA virus; (B) RNA viruses; (C) retroviruses, using reverse transcriptase.

the virus. This process of making proteins on specifications from the DNA via an intermediary RNA is a fundamental biological mechanism of reproduction of all cellular life, from the most simple of bacteria to specialized human cells. Viruses, however, which are vastly simpler life forms than cellular life, possess only DNA or RNA but not both. There are, thus, two kinds of viruses, DNA viruses and RNA viruses. In the case of the DNA viruses the process of protein manufacture follows the same route as with cellular life, i.e. an intermediary messenger RNA is made on a DNA template (although the host cell's machinery is used for the actual manufacture of proteins). In the case of RNA viruses, the RNA genes can themselves, or via another intermediary RNA molecule, direct the manufacture of proteins. However, there is a very important group of viruses that has RNA genes; when the virus enters into cells a DNA copy of the genes (referred to as a provirus) is made, which takes responsibility for the synthesis of proteins. This DNA copy physically integrates into the DNA of the cell to direct the formation of the messenger RNA for the manufacture of the requisite proteins. The key discovery of reverse transcriptase answered a major question in biology of how DNA could be made from an RNA template and earned for its discoverers, Baltimore and Temin, the Nobel prize. Viruses possessing this enzyme, which is unique in nature, are appropriately called retroviruses (the technical name for the family is Retroviridae), and many of them are important causes of virally produced malignant tumours and leukaemias in animals.

The second important discovery on the road to elucidating the cause of

AIDS was made in the laboratory of Robert Gallo at the National Cancer Institute of the National Institutes of Health just outside Washington DC. In 1976 workers under Gallo discovered a growth factor for mature T-lymphocytes which would permit these cells to grow in culture in the laboratory. The lymphocyte is a key cell in the immune system of the body and an important subgroup of lymphocytes are the T-lymphocytes, so-called because their precursors are programmed in infancy to develop into T-lymphocytes by the thymus gland. These lymphocytes serve as regulator cells which modulate the functions of other cells of the immune system and are also executive cells, carrying out some of the cellular effector functions of the immune response. With the ability now available to grow T-lymphocytes in culture came the discovery of a number of viruses which specifically infect lymphocytes, the so-called lymphotropic viruses ('-tropic' denotes the tendency for a virus to infect a particular type of organ, thus neurotropic for viruses infecting nervous tissue, hepatotropic for viruses of the liver, and lymphotropic for lymphocytes).

Following these two important breakthroughs it was not long before the first human retrovirus was isolated from a patient with a leukaemia of the mature T-lymphocytes. The virus was called by Gallo the human T-lymphotropic virus I, abbreviated as HTLV-I, and still remains the only tumour virus definitively established to be a causal agent of a human malignancy. A second virus, HTLV-II, virologically different from HTLV-I, was isolated shortly after, also from a patient with a T-lymphocyte leukaemia, although its causal role in the malignancy had not been established at the time of writing.

The world of tumour virology, and specifically human tumour virology, received an immense boost from these breakthroughs. Another offshoot of these two discoveries that was to have enormously important implications for medical virology, and specifically to the study of viruses and chronic degenerative diseases, was the finding that a group of viruses called slow viruses also belonged to the family of the retroviruses. These viruses, so-called because of the very slow and prolonged nature of the disease they cause, are responsible for degenerative diseases drawn out over years, frequently affecting the central nervous system and progressively and inexorably leading to death. The first of these diseases, described by an Icelandic physician Bjorn Sigurdsson in the 1950s, is due to a virus which causes two separate diseases called, respectively, visna, if the brain is involved, and maedi, if the lungs are affected. The visna-maedi virus caused serious epidemics in sheep in Iceland in the 1940s. A number of related diseases of animals were subsequently described, all characterized by this slow and inexorably fatal course and many of them also affecting the immune system of animals causing immunosuppression. (Studies of these viruses and the mechanisms by which they produce disease have become the basis of a number of research programmes investigating the viral link with a number of chronic degenerative diseases of humans such as multiple sclerosis.) This subgroup of viruses within the retrovirus family were later called lenti-viruses ('lenti' meaning 'slow' in Latin) to distinguish them from the retro-viruses associated with tumours (oncoviruses).

Some retroviruses such as the feline leukaemia virus of cats are known to do both – cause leukaemia as well as a slow type of disease resembling AIDS. Observations of these slow viruses in general, and the feline leukae-mia virus in particular, provided the clues for two groups of workers to attempt to isolate a retrovirus from the T-lymphocytes of AIDS patients. In 1983 Dr Francoise Barré-Sinoussi together with Professor Luc Montagnier, the head of the Viral Cancer Unit of the Pasteur Institute, published a paper in the journal *Science* describing the isolation of a retrovirus from a patient with lymphadenopathy syndrome, one of the disease manifesta-tions which precedes AIDS, and called it the LAV (lymphadenopathy virus) (Fig. 0.3). The following year Dr Robert Gallo's laboratory at the National Institutes of Health became the first laboratory to propagate the virus in cell culture, and he called it HTLV-III (to follow on from the earlier human T-lymphotropic retroviruses isolated in his laboratory). The virus was sub-sequently given the rather cumbersome name of HTLV-III/LAV to provide equal recognition to both scientific groups. To compound the confusion, a virus isolated from an AIDS patient by Dr Jay Levy of the University of California, soon after Gallo's first isolation, was given yet another name, ARV (for AIDS-related virus).

Unfortunately the nomenclature issue became but a relatively minor aspect of what was soon to develop into a monumental dispute of international proportions which was only settled, albeit temporarily, by a formal agree-ment between the then Presidents Reagan of the USA and Mitterand of France, which gave equal recognition to both workers. Not only was indi-vidual and parochial prestige involved in claiming credit for the discovery of the viral cause of AIDS but, in addition, vast financial interests were implicated in the marketing of diagnostic tests based on the isolated viruses. The acrimonious dispute was renewed in 1990 when Pasteur Institute scientists decided to analyse the genetic structure of Gallo's virus and compare it with that of Montagnier's initial isolate. They showed them to be so similar that it was very unlikely that they were not one and the same virus. (Some differences in genetic structure are expected between virus

Isolation of a T-Lymphotropic Retrovirus from a Patient at Risk for Acquired Immune Deficiency Syndrome (AIDS)

Abstract. *A retrovirus belonging to the family of recently discovered human T-cell leukemia viruses (HTLV), but clearly distinct from each previous isolate, has been isolated from a Caucasian patient with signs and symptoms that often precede the acquired immune deficiency syndrome (AIDS). This virus is a typical type-C RNA tumor virus, buds from the cell membrane, prefers magnesium for reverse transcriptase activity, and has an internal antigen (p25) similar to HTLV p24. Antibodies from serum of this patient react with proteins from viruses of the HTLV-I subgroup, but type-specific antisera to HTLV-I do not precipitate proteins of the new isolate. The virus from this patient has been transmitted into cord blood lymphocytes, and the virus produced by these cells is similar to the original isolate. From these studies it is concluded that this virus as well as the previous HTLV isolates belong to a general family of T-lymphotropic retroviruses that are horizontally transmitted in humans and may be involved in several pathological syndromes, including AIDS.*

Fig 0.3 Report in Science, 20 May 1983, by F. Barré-Sinoussi and others in the laboratories of Dr Luc Montagnier, announcing the isolation of a retrovirus associated with the development of AIDS.

isolates taken from different patients and, in the case of the retroviruses which mutate so frequently, even isolates taken from the same patient at different times, although these would only be fairly subtle differences.) Rather uncomfortably for Gallo, Montagnier had, in fact, sent his original isolates to Gallo in the course of customary scientific exchange in September 1983, soon after the Frenchman made his first isolation. Fortunately, however, the revival of the quarrel was quashed when it was admitted from Montagnier's laboratory that there had been contamination of strains. Montagnier's original LAV isolate codenamed Bru (after the first three letters of the patient's surname) had been contaminated some months later by another faster growing strain codenamed Lai, and this strain he had inadvertently sent to Gallo, which in turn inadvertently contaminated Gallo's cultures. It has now generally been accepted that credit should be shared between the two – Montagnier for the original isolation and Gallo for the ability to propagate the virus and to develop the critically needed diagnostic tests. By international convention a neutral name has been chosen for the virus, that of human immunodeficiency virus or HIV.

With the development of diagnostic tests for the virus came the ability to define its extent and chart its behaviour in human populations far more accurately than the clinical definition alone could do. A particularly important aspect of infection with HIV was the demonstration that individuals presenting clinically with AIDS merely accounted for a very small visible proportion of all those infected with the virus. A far larger number of people were infected but had not yet reached the stage where they clinically manifested the disease. By studying these so-called asymptomatically infected individuals and closely following them over time it became evident that this silent phase could last for many years before the disease of AIDS manifested itself. This long period of silent infection with a chronic, inexorably fatal course fitted in well with the characteristic features of other slow virus diseases.

In 1986 a second HIV virus was isolated by Luc Montagnier's group from AIDS patients in Guinea Bissau and the Cape Verde Islands, and was called LAV-2. At about the same time an American group under Myron Essex also isolated in neighbouring Senegal a second virus which they called HTLV-IV. Although the French–American dispute initially prevented a comparison of these two viruses, it was subsequently shown to be the same virus and was called HIV-2.

Following the discovery of the viral cause of AIDS, research into the development of drugs that act on the virus could take off. A particular antiretroviral agent from the past, called azido-thymidine (AZT), which had been used some decades before to effectively treat experimental retrovirus infection in laboratory mice, became one of the most important specific therapies for AIDS patients. The availability of the causative virus also ushered in a gigantic research effort to develop a specific vaccine.

After the rapid research advances of the 1980s, progress in the early 1990s appeared to stall somewhat for a few years. A despondency set in with a widespread feeling amongst healthcare workers and researchers that medical science would be unable to effectively control this seemingly relentlessly progressive infectious disease. The antiretroviral drugs that were available at that time, mainly AZT and two or three other nucleoside analogues, were only temporarily effective as HIV ultimately became resistant to them. Added to these setbacks in drug therapy were the failures of the early HIV vaccine trials in experimental animals. The prevailing feeling was that HIV infection meant inevitable death.

The mid-to-late 1990s, however, witnessed a gratifying turn-around. Advances in antiretroviral therapy, significant progress towards the development of HIV/AIDS vaccines and a fundamental change in perceptions of how the virus multiplies and produces disease all contributed to a great deal more optimism for managing the infection. Diagnostic tests to accurately quantitate the amount of virus in the bloodstream became part of routine clinical management and provided the means to closely monitor the effects of treatment and to predict prognosis with reasonable confidence. The therapeutic goal in treating HIV infection was now recognized to be to directly reduce the amount of virus in the body by antiretroviral drugs. Single-drug therapy (monotherapy) was replaced by multidrug combinations using two or three antiretroviral drugs given simultaneously, thereby greatly reducing the chances of the virus developing resistance. Combination drug therapy, often referred to as HAART (highly active antiretroviral therapy), became the beacon of hope to HIV-infected persons and it now appeared that they could lead normal lives with good immune function for an indefinite period of time as long as they were able to tolerate the therapy and could afford to pay for it.

Unfortunately, however, the enormous cost of combination antiretroviral therapy essentially precludes its availability for the developing world where by far the majority of HIV-infected persons live. In the late 1990s there is still a great deal of pessimism regarding the failure to effectively control the spread of HIV infection by changing lifestyle habits and attitudes towards safer sexual practices, particularly in the developing world. Ultimately, the control of the epidemic worldwide remains the development of an effective vaccine and significant progress does appear to have been made towards realizing this goal.

Despite the overwhelming evidence establishing HIV as the cause of AIDS, a very small number of scientists have persisted to this day in sowing unnecessary confusion in the minds of the uninformed by disputing the role of HIV in AIDS. Foremost among these has been Dr Peter Duesberg, a molecular virologist at the University of Berkeley that HIV does not play a direct causal role in AIDS but is merely present as a 'passenger' virus. This hypothesis has found little suppport amongst serious HIV researchers and, unfortunately, a consderable amount of resources have had to be expended in rebutting these 'theories' and attempting to clarify the confusion and the potential damage that they have caused.

The origins of AIDS

Given the intense and unique social, political and human implications of AIDS, it is small wonder that questions surrounding the origins of this remarkable virus and its equally remarkable disease have fired the imagination ever since it was first recognized. Is AIDS a new or old disease? Did it first arise in Africa or in the USA? Where did the virus come from? These questions have been debated and argued over at great depth in scientific and lay forums alike and still arouse considerable controversy. In reality the answers to these questions, if they are ever forthcoming, will have little relevance to the control or management of the disease. In fact, little is known about the origins of any human virus, let alone HIV. Nevertheless, the drive and curiosity to search for answers to these tantalizing questions has prompted a great deal of investigative research as well as wide-ranging speculation. What is incontestable is that the disease of AIDS was first recognized in the USA and only somewhat later was the epidemic as such observed in Europe and the African continent. However, various scenarios of the birth and development of the epidemic have been built around pieces of knowledge recruited from a number of diverse sources. At present the answers to both the origin of the disease as well as to the ancestry of the virus remain as unresolved as when the questions were first posed.

In essence, three conjectural accounts of the natural history of the AIDS epidemic have been put forward, two of them pointing to the African continent for the origin of the virus. One of the earliest of these postulates, published in 1984 – a year after the African connection was uncovered by Belgian and French workers – holds that the disease of AIDS is not a new disease but is rather one of the old endemic diseases of Africa which has been, hitherto, silent or unrecognized. That the infection could have existed undetected in humans for centuries should not be particularly surprising as laboratory diagnostic facilities in many African countries are still poor or virtually non-existent. Clinical illnesses with fever in Africa are usually ascribed to malaria, and pneumonia to tuberculosis, without any further investigations taking place. Over the past few decades a number of formidable viral diseases, and in particular the African viral haemorrhagic fevers, have suddenly made dramatic appearances in humans causing acute, virulent and often fatal illnesses. The origins of two of these diseases, Marburg and Ebola viral haemorrhagic fevers, are still shrouded in mystery, while others, such as Lassa fever, have been demonstrated to have long been endemic in African populations, causing silent infections in most Africans and the dreaded haemorrhagic fever disease usually in non-African expatriates. Similarly, a number of viral infections which have been in Europe for centuries, such as smallpox and measles, caused devastating epidemics when they were introduced into African populations in the eighteenth and nineteenth centuries (see Chapter 10). Thus, HIV could also have been an endemic virus, present for centuries in central Africa, and contained by the sparse contact with outsiders until political developments in Africa, together with the revolution in regional and international travel, broadened the ecological niche of the virus and introduced it into Western countries. Here the spread was facilitated by the sexual revolution and the widespread use of the hollow-bore needle for illicit intravenous drug administration.

Against the theory that AIDS is an age-old endemic disease of Africa is the difficulty that many investigators have encountered in trying to find evidence of infection with HIV in stored serum specimens of populations in various parts of Africa before the 1980s. Some of the earlier studies that did find samples of sera with a high prevalence of HIV antibodies misled workers into believing that this was confirmatory evidence for the long-standing endemicity of HIV in Africa. However, these high rates of anti-body positivity, we now know, are probably due to technical factors and in particular the sera of African subjects often contain substantial levels of globulin proteins which can interfere with serological testing and give false-positive results – the so-called 'stickiness' of African sera. Modern testing of archived African sera is, in fact, rarely positive and this suggests that HIV infection could not have been responsible for anything more than the relatively rare infections before the 1980s. This is also corroborated by reports of doctors with many years of clinical experience in developing Africa, who have quite categorically denied having seen diseases resembling AIDS in the past. Clinical signs of AIDS are usually so strikingly characteristic that it would have been most unlikely that a whole epidemic could have been missed.

The evidence is therefore very much stronger that the virus is indeed new in humans, possibly having been introduced into the human population in the 1950s. The earliest serum specimen retrieved from archived frozen material, shown to be positive for HIV antibodies, was taken from a patient in 1959 in Kinshasha in the then Belgian Congo (now the Democratic Republic of the Congo). No material before that time has yet been shown to have HIV antibodies. Also, given the rapid spread of infection which has been observed throughout the world since 1980, it is hardly likely that this virus could have circulated in Man much before the 1950s and still have been unrecognized.

The second postulated scenario holds that the human virus originated from the monkey immunodeficiency virus, or, as it is more scientifically correctly called, the simian immunodeficiency virus or SIV. There are, in fact, a number of SIV strains, each one specific to the monkey species that it infects. Thus we have SIVagm which infects the African green monkey (or vervet monkey), the SIVmnd of the mandrill ape, SIVsm of the sooty mangabey monkey, and others. Each strain will, under natural conditions, infect only its specific species of monkey and, similarly, no SIV will infect humans. HIV also cannot infect any animal other than humans except under experimental laboratory conditions where infection can be induced in chimpanzees (although it apparently does not cause disease in this animal). There are also immunodeficiency viruses in other animals; for example, cats, cattle, horses, sheep and goats and, again, natural infections with each of these viruses will only occur in their specific host animal. By examining the nucleotide (the building blocks of the nucleic acid of the virus) sequences of the genetic material of these different viruses, the extent of similarities and differences between them can be calculated and a family tree of their relative relatedness can be drawn up. What is of interest is that the evolutionary tree of these immunodeficiency viruses parallels the evolutionary development of the animal species that they infect. Thus the closest relative of HIV is SIV. This evolutionary relationship is not unique to immunodeficiency viruses but has also been demonstrated with other viruses such as the herpes virus family.

Within the SIV group of viruses the sooty mangabey virus (SIVsm) shows the closest relationship to an HIV strain, in fact HIV-2. The geographical distribution of the HIV-2 virus is quite remarkable in that it appears to be relatively confined to West African countries and also the former Portuguese colonies of Angola and Mozambique. In these countries HIV-2 is generally more common than HIV-1. It is of interest that the natural habitat of the sooty mangabey monkey is also the forests of West Africa. Furthermore, the genetic sequence relationship between SIVsm and HIV-2 is as close as that between different isolates of SIVsm themselves. However, there still remains a question mark over the link between HIV-1 and SIV. This missing link may have been discovered by the recent isolation of a virus from a captive chimpanzee in Gabon in 1989, and now called SIVcpz. This virus is far more closely related to HIV-1 than any other immunodeficiency virus and is also the only virus that possesses the same set of genes as HIV-1. The link should, however, still be treated with some reserve as there has as yet only been one single isolate, and that in a captive animal. It is still possible that SIVcpz could be a human virus which for some unknown reason infected that particular chimpanzee.

As fascinating as this genetic detective work is, the question still remains as to how simian viruses, whether they be SIVsm or SIVcpz, could have jumped the species barrier to become HIV-2 and HIV-1 respectively. One would still need to postulate that a mutation, or more likely a sequence of mutations, occurred in the simian virus to enable it to infect humans. Amongst virologists it is well known that RNA viruses in general and the retroviruses in particular do mutate at a very high rate. One would also need to postulate some mechanism by which a virus that is of low infectivity and is transmissible only by intimate contact could have been physically transmitted from monkey to humans. Monkeys do form a source of protein for humans in certain parts of tropical Africa and it is feasible that in the process of hunting and capturing these animals, blood from monkeys could have entered into the bloodstream of humans via abrasions or skin wounds or defects in the oral mucous membrane. Another possibility that has been offered is that chimpanzee and monkey blood, which has been used in years gone past for malaria research, could have been the conduit into the human species. Outlandish suggestions have also been forthcoming of supposed tribal rituals involving the splashing of monkey blood over human genital organs to enhance sexual performance or sexual intercourse with monkeys as the possible route.

More recently allegations have been made incriminating early oral polio vaccines as the source of SIV infection of humans with its subsequent mutation to HIV. Early trials of oral polio vaccines in the late 1950s were carried out by spraying prototype vaccines into the mouth and throat of several hundred thousand people in Rwanda, Zaire and Burundi, precisely the early epicentres of the AIDS epidemic in Africa.

Oral polio vaccine consists of a suspension of live vaccine strains of poliovirus and certainly the initial production lots of vaccine were not tested for contaminating simian viruses. These vaccines are produced on cell cultures derived from monkey kidneys and those coming from the African green monkey (which is still one of the most commonly used cell culture systems for oral polio vaccine) could well have been contaminated with SIVagm. However, there is at yet no evidence that even HIV can be contracted from ingesting contaminated material other than the rare reported cases of HIV transmitted via oral sex or to infants from breast feeding.

An alternate 'hypothesis' relates to the common use of oral polio vaccine to treat cold sores (herpes simplex) on the lips or genital organs, a practice common amongst homosexual men. This could, in theory, have afforded the opportunity for any contaminating SIVagm to have been inoculated through the skin barrier giving it the potential of reaching receptive cells to infect.

There is, however, little scientific substance to these 'hypotheses'. The genetic differences between SIVagm and HIV-1 are so vast, in fact the two viruses do not even have all their genes in common, that it would be scientifically quite impossible to conceive how SIVagm could have been able to establish infection given our knowledge of HIV transmissibility and then, furthermore, to have undergone such vast genetic changes to become HIV within a few years. There is much concern in scientific and public health circles that, even though the biological absurdity of these propositions is apparent, they may still cause untold harm to immunization programmes such as the global programme to eradicate polio.

The postulated sequence of events with all these 'hypotheses' thus relates mutations in monkey virus (SIVsm or SIVcpz or a related strain) leading to a crossing of the species barrier and to infection of humans in Africa followed by the subsequent introduction into the Western world where its spread was accelerated by the sexual revolution and use of the hollow-bore needle. This hypothesis has support from observations of the first known appearances of the disease in various parts of the world. As already mentioned, the first laboratory demonstration of human infection by detection of antibodies was from an archived serum specimen taken in 1959 in Zaire. The first isolation of the virus also came from an archived serum specimen from Central Africa collected in 1976. A number of cases of AIDS-like diseases were reported in Central Africa among foreigners and locals in 1976 and 1977, including the well-publicized case of a Danish woman who had apparently acquired the infection while working as a surgeon in Zaire in 1976 and who subsequently died the following year. Towards the end of the 1970s and the beginning of the 1980s, AIDS cases were observed on the island of Haiti and amongst Haitians living in the USA; indeed, Haiti was assumed to be the link between the African continent and the USA as it has long been a favourite holiday playground for homosexual men from the USA. There is, however, evidence that the advent of AIDS in the USA may well have predated that in Haiti – the earliest observed AIDS-like disease in the USA was reported to have occurred in 1968 in a 15-year-old sexually active boy. The route of the virus may well have been the reverse, from the USA to Haiti. In any event the mid-1970s saw increasing tourist contacts between the USA and Africa and the virus is far more likely to have been introduced directly into the USA from Africa.

The third viewpoint on the origin of AIDS and HIV is one based largely on more general observations of the global AIDS epidemic and is probably the one that is closest to the truth. There is little doubt that the epidemic of AIDS began in humans in the late seventies and early eighties and has increased in extent since then. The odd isolated case of AIDS-like disease before then was probably of little relevance either in Africa or in the USA, and does not alter the broader notion of an almost simultaneous appearance and spread of the epidemic in the USA, Europe and Africa. Supporting this theory are studies of sera taken from populations both in the USA and in Africa which have revealed very low prevalences of infections with HIV before that time. This contrasts dramatically with the picture towards the end of the 1980s of a disease with a high prevalence in certain high-risk groups, and a fairly rapidly spreading epidemic.

The dimensions of the fearsomeness of AIDS

The AIDS epidemic has in many ways been a humbling experience to medical science. Its advent at the closing of the twentieth century, a century that has seen technology progressively and purposefully overcome so many human diseases, has indeed given cause for reflection on the true limitations of what may previously have been thought to be the almost limitless achievements and accomplishments of humans. AIDS has probably now become one of the most formidable of all diseases in human history. In terms of death and illness it is true that AIDS falls well short of the great plague which killed a quarter of Europe's population in the Middle Ages, or even the great Spanish influenza pandemic which killed 20 million people at the close of the first World War – more than were killed in that 'great war to end all wars'. However, AIDS has four cardinal features which together make it a uniquely formidable disease. Firstly that it is infectious and transmissible from person to person. Secondly, that once infection occurs it follows an inexorable course to disease and eventually to death in most, if not all, cases. Thirdly, that all persons infected with HIV apparently remain infectious; that is they are able to transmit the virus to others to a greater or lesser extent, for the rest of their lives. Fourthly, that the reservoir of infection, that is the total sum of people infected who can also act as a source of infectious virus to others, is constantly and progressively expanding as the epidemic spreads to involve more and more individuals.

Compounding the terror generated by this disease even further are its social, psychological and political dimensions. In Western countries AIDS has largely affected groups who have been to a lesser or greater extent victimized, ostracized and marginalized by the rest of society – homosexual men, especially with the association of promiscuity and perverse practices in communal bathhouses, and intravenous drug users, individuals who have been viewed as derelicts of society. To a lesser extent in Third World countries, female prostitutes have been marginalized by their respective societies. This association of societal rejection, together with a morbid dread of acquiring infection, has given rise to unique feelings of revulsion and condemnation of victims of the disease. It has renewed the ugliness of people's feelings towards their fellows and revitalized homophobia, 'gay bashing' and naked racism. It has given reactionary politicians ammunition to advocate, and in some instances even implement, restrictive legislation on the pretext of the good of the community taking precedence over the rights of the individual. In the medical and nursing professions fear has, in many cases, profoundly affected the code of ethical practice of these professions.

As discussed above and as will become apparent in the forthcoming chapters of this book, AIDS is a new and unique disease. It is new to scientists, it is new to doctors, it is new to psychologists and social workers, it is new to theologians and ethicists and it is new to legal experts and politicians. We are still in the learning curve but much has been learnt, and the knowledge and experience gained has, and will, change the practice of medicine from here onwards.

1

What is AIDS and how does it manifest itself?

Some AIDS definitions

'AIDS' has now become, by common usage, a word in the English language, as has 'SIDA' in the French language and similarly other foreign language equivalents. On an emotional level, the meaning of AIDS scarcely needs elaborating. Few people have not heard the word and to many it conveys a very striking image of a skeletal body and a cadaver-like open-mouthed face of a terminal patient.

As mentioned in the Introduction, AIDS is the acronym for 'acquired immunodeficiency syndrome' and was a term coined early on in the history of the disease. AIDS is, by definition, the end-stage disease manifestation of an infection with a virus called the human immunodeficiency virus (HIV). The virus infects mainly two systems of the body, the immune system and the central nervous system, and disease manifestations are consequent on damage to these two systems.

Much store is set and a great deal of fuss is made by counsellors and educationalists in the field of AIDS in emphasizing the distinction between infection with the virus and the disease of AIDS. The distinction is a very simple and straightforward one and is based on an appreciation that HIV, like many other viruses, can infect the body and multiply in many cells inside the body without causing any ostensible damage, that is damage of which the patient is aware. In this respect HIV is not unique. The herpes viruses, for example, do this. Herpes simplex virus usually first infects human beings in infancy, often causing blisters, ulcers and marked inflammation and pain in the mouth, lips, gums and tongue and producing a feverish, fretful and highly irritable baby (often being daubed with soothing gentian violet around the mouth). When the infant recovers the sores heal and the inflammation subsides, and the episode is often soon forgotten. However, the virus has not been eliminated but remains behind and persists in the body in the form of a silent or latent infection in nervous tissue. Here it can exist for a lifetime causing no harm but multiplying at such a low rate that the person is unaware that they still harbour the virus. However, on occasions, some triggering episode may occur in the individual, a fever due to infections or psychological stress or suppression of the immune system, which will bring the virus out of its latent state and cause it to multiply rapidly. It then travels down a nerve to reach the skin and mucous membrane of the lips and mouth where it causes 'fever blisters' or 'cold sores'. These will heal and the episode may then be repeated cyclically at intervals.

There are also several other examples of viruses that cause silent infections without any clinical signs or symptoms – sometimes permanently so that the individual is never aware of their infection unless laboratory tests are done to demonstrate the presence of the virus. Sometimes they can manifest clinically at a later stage when the virus is activated.

The HIV virus shares with herpes virus this tendency to cause silent infections. When it first infects, it may or may not cause clinical disease, as will be seen later in the chapter, but soon settles into its latent or silent phase which usually lasts for many years. At the later stages of its natural history, the virus enters into a phase where it actively multiplies to a far greater degree and then produces disease manifestations. The first clinical signs and symptoms are not specific for AIDS but later on they do progress to the typical clinical presentation of AIDS.

HIV infection and AIDS thus really refer to two different aspects of the same process. An individual with HIV infection has thus been infected with the HIV virus which is established and replicating in the cells of his or her body, and the infection may be in a silent phase or it may cause disease manifestations, depending on the stage of its natural history. If it is causing disease and the disease manifestations fit into the definition of AIDS, we would then diagnose that individual as having AIDS (due, of course, to HIV infection). Thus, to return to the original definition, AIDS is the end-stage disease manifestation of HIV infection. HIV infection may or may not clinically manifest itself as the disease AIDS depending on the stage of its natural history in that individual.

Another issue of terminology which causes some consternation is whether the term AIDS virus is permissible as an alternative to HIV. There are many who feel that AIDS virus should not be used as AIDS occurs in only a small minority of individuals infected with the virus. Undoubtedly, compassion for individuals who are infected and the harsh implications that go along with the term AIDS virus dictate that one should, where possible, avoid the more emotive terminology for the virus. Certainly HIV is the scientifically accepted designation. However, the term AIDS virus is not intrinsically or scientifically incorrect, merely referring to the virus which is the causal agent of the AIDS disease. There are many viruses that are designated by the name of the disease that they are capable of causing, even though the disease manifestation may not always be a consequence of infection. For example, mumps virus may infect but cause no clinically apparent disease in up to a third of individuals. Poliovirus only causes poliomyelitis in less than 1% of individuals infected by that virus.

'Western AIDS' and 'African AIDS'

Soon after the discovery of the extensive epidemic of HIV infection in Africa in 1983 it became apparent that the characteristics of the epidemic in that part of the world differed quite markedly from the characteristics of that in Western countries but with a number of clearly defined clinical differences. The distinction between Western AIDS and African AIDS, as the two forms of the disease became known, was based primarily on epidemiological differences, especially with regard to the groups of people within the population who were mainly affected and also how the virus was predominantly transmitted. These terms have now, to some extent, become obsolete and the so-called African pattern of AIDS is certainly not confined to Africa. The term African AIDS also has come to take on a somewhat pejorative connotation.

In 1988 the WHO proposed that the global epidemiology of AIDS be divided into three patterns. Pattern 1 is the pattern of AIDS found in North America, in Western Europe and in Australia and New Zealand. In these countries the sexual transmission of HIV virus is mainly by homosexual intercourse and HIV infection is predominantly found in homosexual and bisexual men. Transmission by contaminated blood transfusions has dropped dramatically with the advent of routine screening of blood, but sharing of needles for intravenous drug abuse has become the second most important route of transmission. The ratio of males to females is greatly in favour of males, up to 20 to 1 in some pattern 1 countries, due to the prevalence of the disease in homosexual men. Because of the relatively low numbers of women involved, paediatric infection is very low in these countries. Thus, an essential component of the pattern 1 HIV epidemiology is that infection is concentrated in so-called high-risk groups, mainly homosexual and bisexual men and intravenous drug abusers, where the prevalence of infection may be up to 50% or more. However, in the rest of the population infection is uncommon; for example, the prevalence of HIV in prospective blood donors (a population group where the prevalence of infection is easy to measure because of routine screening), the prevalence of HIV is usually less than 0.1% in most pattern 1 countries.

Pattern 2 is that found in sub-Saharan Africa, Central America and also the inner city populations living in deprived socio-economic communities in the big cities of the USA. Infection there is predominantly transmitted by heterosexual intercourse with males and females being affected almost equally or, if anything, with a slight predominance in females. The adult males infected are usually somewhat older than the adult females, as is characteristically seen with other sexually transmitted diseases. The traditional 'high-risk' groups seen in pattern 1 regions are of little or no importance in pattern 2 regions, and no clear-cut 'high-risk' groups can be defined other than highly promiscuous individuals such as female prostitutes or those in occupations where sexual promiscuity is rife, for example long-distance truck drivers. Infection tends to be more common in the urban rather than rural populations. In many large African cities infection may reach up to 30% of all adults, and in female prostitutes up to 90%. Blood-borne transmission plays proportionately a far lesser role than sexual transmission even though, in many African countries, screening of blood is often deficient or sometimes even absent and also re-use of unsterile needles for injection or for tribal scarification practices contributes significantly to HIV transmission. Intravenous drug abuse, however, is rare in Africa. Because of the large number of women infected with the virus, paediatric AIDS is a sizeable problem in pattern 2 regions, being responsible for up to 15% or more of all AIDS cases there.

The term pattern 3 AIDS is used for regions where the virus has been introduced at a much later stage than in pattern 1 and 2 regions and has, as yet, not become fully established. However, as the disease continues to progress globally, and as recent political developments speed up contacts with many of these countries which were previously isolated from Western vices and virtues, so has the extent of this privileged pattern 3 group shrunk. Originally pattern 3 regions included North Africa, the Middle East, Eastern Europe, Asia and the Pacific. HIV infection was comparatively rare in most countries in these regions and was essentially confined to foreigners, prostitutes and intravenous drug abusers. However, in a number of these erstwhile pattern 3 regions, for example Thailand and

India, the global advance of the epidemic has radically changed this, and in both countries the infection rate has increased alarmingly in recent times. Nevertheless, some countries such as China, which houses approximately a quarter of the world's population, still reported (as at July 1997) only 155 cases out of a worldwide total of 1 736 958 (November 1997).

The division of the global epidemiology of AIDS into these three patterns is, of course, merely arbitrary for the sake of convenience. Within many countries features of both pattern 1 and pattern 2 exist side by side; for example, the USA, which is essentially a pattern 1 country, has largely a type 2 pattern in its inner city populations. In South Africa the AIDS epidemic began with pattern 1 characteristics, predominantly in the higher socio-economic white population, affecting mainly homosexual men. The first reported case of AIDS in a black person in 1987 heralded the beginning of a pattern 2 epidemic which a few years ago overtook pattern 1 and is now by far the dominant pattern in that country. Nevertheless, this division does serve a useful function in promoting the understanding of the dynamics of the epidemic in a particular population, and does provide a rational basis to focus appropriate educational and other interventions, which will be discussed later.

The components of AIDS

In the introductory chapter the reason why most viruses specifically infect a particular species of animal was discussed. Thus very few animal viruses are able to infect humans and, likewise, most human viruses can only infect animals under experimental conditions and often with great difficulty or not at all. Also discussed was how, even within the realm of human viruses, certain specific organs of the body would be infected by specific viruses, a feature called tropism. In the case of HIV there are mainly two organ systems for which the virus has a specific tropism – the cells of the immune system, because of the presence of specific receptor sites for HIV on these cells (which will be discussed in detail in Chapter 3), and also the cells of the nervous system, although it is not clear precisely which receptor sites are involved here.

In the immune system of the body there are two main types of cells that are infected by HIV: firstly, the lymphocytes, and specifically the T-helper or CD4 lymphocytes, which function as the regulator cells for the immune system and thus play a central role in the control of immune function; secondly, cells called monocytes and macrophages whose function it is to rid the body of foreign proteins by ingesting them and also to present them to the immune system to enable an immune response to be mounted against them. Monocytes and macrophages are not destroyed by being infected with HIV but, as we will see in Chapter 3, their importance with regard to HIV infection lies in the fact that the virus can replicate in these cells without apparently harming them, and they thus act as the major reservoir for infectious virus in the body. The effect of HIV infection on the T-helper lymphocyte is quite devastating and results in profound depletion of these cells – the hallmark of HIV-related disease. The striking loss of these key cells of the immune system results in a profound suppression of immune function. No other infectious agent causes such a severe collapse of the immune system. As a result of this immunosuppression there are two consequences in the body. Firstly, there are the effects that are directly due to extreme immunosuppression and that can be reproduced in experimental animals; for example, by artificially suppressing the immune system of laboratory mice with drugs or by surgically removing the thymus gland and causing the development of a syndrome called runting disease. Similar elements of runting disease in mice are seen in humans with severe immunosuppression. There is a profound weight loss, in severe cases individuals may lose up to 50% of their body weight in six months (in East Africa a common name for AIDS is 'slim disease'). In addition, chronic diarrhoea (sometimes called 'wet AIDS'), which may persist for many months, and also a chronically elevated body temperature or pyrexia (also called 'hot AIDS') may also be continually present for prolonged periods of time. Another direct effect of HIV on the immune system is enlargement and swelling of lymph glands; this is called lymphadenopathy and is one of the first of the clinical manifestations of HIV infection.

The indirect effects of immunosuppression are responsible for perhaps the more prominent clinical manifestations of AIDS and are also the most common causes of death. The disabling of the immune system renders the body vulnerable to infections with a large variety of micro-organisms, as well as the development of malignant tumours. In general, three kinds of infectious agents may assail the body. Firstly, there are micro-organisms, especially viruses that affect healthy and immunosuppressed individuals alike. In normal individuals these organisms can cause acute but temporary illness, as an intact immune system is readily able to deal with them. However, immunosuppressed persons will usually suffer from these infections to a more severe and often more prolonged extent. Secondly, there are organisms, particularly bacteria, fungi and parasitic organisms, that in normal individuals produce disease but are usually readily dealt with by antimicrobial drugs and antibiotics. With immunosuppressed individuals, treatment of these infections is often difficult because of the absence of auxiliary help from the immune system, and these organisms, because they persist for prolonged periods of time, often develop resistance to the anti-microbial drugs. Thirdly, there are infections with organisms that are of low virulence in healthy individuals and seldom cause any disease manifestations or at most relatively trivial infections. Many of these organisms are present for long periods of time or are even permanently in the body, but are prevented from causing disease by an intact immune system. It is these micro-organisms which cause the infectious diseases that are characteristic of immunosuppressed individuals in general and in AIDS in particular. They are commonly referred to as opportunistic infections.

Opportunistic infections are caused by organisms throughout the micro-biological spectrum – viruses, bacteria, fungi and parasites. Amongst the more commonly involved viruses is cytomegalovirus (CMV), a common inhabitant of the human body in healthy as well as immunosuppressed individuals. In AIDS patients CMV is a common cause of severe pneumonia which is often lethal. It may also infect the retina of the eye and is a frequent cause of blindness in these patients. The gastro-intestinal tract is also a common target for the virus where it infects predominantly the colon causing a severe form of colitis, manifesting as abdominal pain and diarrhoea. Herpes simplex virus, usually silent in healthy persons with the occasional short episode of fever blisters (cold sores), may cause, in AIDS patients, severe infections of the skin and mucous membranes and even various internal organs. Shingles due to the varicella zoster virus [which causes both chickenpox (varicella) and shingles (zoster)] is another example of a herpes virus which causes silent infection between the initial bout of chickenpox and the later reactivation of shingles. In AIDS patients severe shingles, which is usually recurrent (in healthy persons shingles usually only occurs once in a lifetime), is a common manifestation of AIDS especially in African patients.

With regard to the opportunistic bacterial infections it is now tuberculosis (caused by *Mycobacterium tuberculosis*) that has become the most important single micro-organism to indicate the onset of AIDS in pattern 2 populations (Fig. 1.1). Although pneumonia is most commonly associated with tuberculosis, in AIDS patients tuberculous disease may often involve organs other than the lungs; for example, tuberculous meningitis and tuberculous lesions in the brain, bone, liver, kidney and other organs. A particularly worrying consequence of the emergence of tuberculosis in HIV-infected persons is the recently observed development of bacteria that are resistant to many of the drugs used for the treatment or prevention of

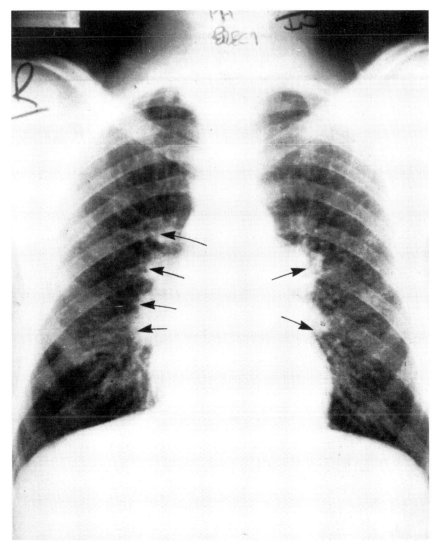

Fig. 1.1 Pulmonary (miliary) tuberculosis in an AIDS patient with diffuse involvement of both lungs and also associated enlargement of (hilar) lymph glands (arrowed). (Photograph courtesy of Dr D C Spencer.)

tuberculosis. These multiresistant strains have caused severe disease in AIDS patients and have spread in the hospital setting to other patients and to health care personnel and have serious public health implications. Bacteria called atypical mycobacteria (related to *Mycobacterium tuberculosis* but

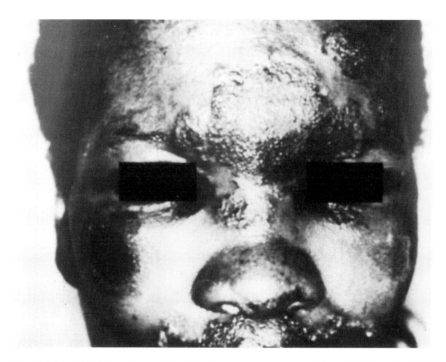

Fig. 1.2 Facial lesions due to *Candida* in a young woman with AIDS who also had involvement of the oral and vaginal mucous membranes. (Photograph courtesy of Dr D C Spencer.)

often resistant to antituberculous drugs) were one of the earliest of the opportunistic infections observed in Western countries and were responsible for most pulmonary disease and occasionally extrapulmonary disease. A variety of other severe bacterial infections may also be part of AIDS, such as septicaemia (bacterial infection of the blood), especially with organisms such as salmonella (a bacterium related to the typhoid bacterium).

A number of fungal organisms are associated with AIDS patients. Thrush (caused by the common fungus *Candida albicans*) is seen in a severe form in AIDS patients (Fig. 1.2), where it may cause extensive lesions of the mouth and other mucous membranes and may be difficult to treat. Another infectious fungal agent, cryptococcus, which is commonly found in soil, may occasionally cause infections by being breathed into the respiratory tract, although it is generally associated with meningitis. In AIDS patients the organism may also cause infections in a number of other organ systems.

The major parasitic infection associated with AIDS, and one which is also the most important single opportunistic micro-organism in pattern 1

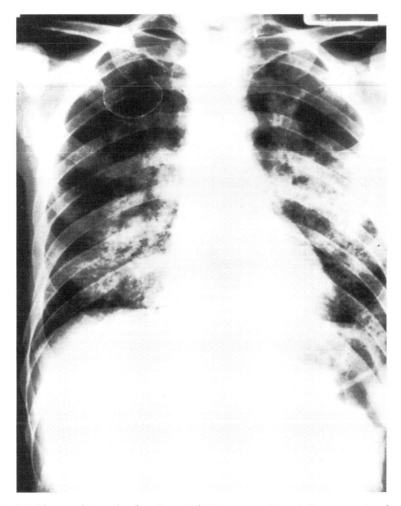

Fig. 1.3 Chest radiograph of patient with *Pneumocystis carinii* pneumonia, showing characteristic fine, patchy, shadowing in both lungs. (Photograph courtesy of
Dr D C Spencer.)

regions, is the parasite *Pneumocystis carinii*, which causes severe pneumonia, often abbreviated to PCP (*Pneumocystis carinii* pneumonia) and
is a frequent cause of death in AIDS patients (Fig. 1.3). This organism
exists in the lungs and respiratory tracts of many healthy individuals
without causing any harm. However, it has now become one of the most
feared of the opportunistic infections in immunosuppressed patients and
especially in AIDS. Related to *Pneumocystis carinii* is another parasite

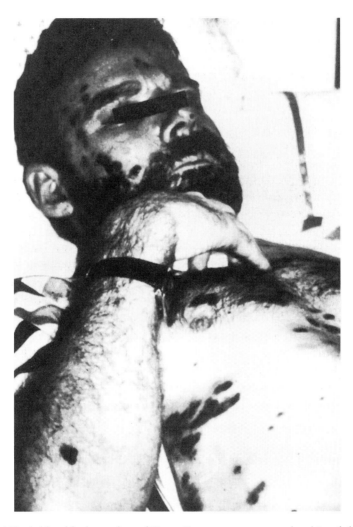

Fig. 1.4 Dark blue-black patches of Kaposi's sarcoma seen on the skin of the face, arm and chest in a patient with AIDS. Lesions are often also found in internal organs in AIDS patients. (Photograph courtesy of Dr D C Spencer.)

called *Toxoplasma gondii* which also seldom causes severe disease in healthy individuals; occasionally it may cause a mild glandular-fever-like illness, especially in persons coming into contact with cats (which are the major hosts of this organism). Various lesions may be caused by toxoplasma but the most important disease manifestation in AIDS patients is its involvement with the brain. Another organism – called *Cryptosporidium*, which had barely been heard of by the majority of medical practitioners before the AIDS era – has now become an important cause of severe chronic diarrhoea in AIDS patients.

A number of malignancies may also act as indicators of AIDS. Kaposi's sarcoma, a disease found in elderly individuals especially men and particularly of Mediterranean and Jewish origin, had been known to cause slow-growing tumours on the skin but very seldom involved internal organs or caused serious disease or death. It had also been observed in Africa but mainly in younger persons. However, among immunosuppressed individuals, and now especially noticed in AIDS patients particularly homosexual men, a more fast growing and aggressive Kaposi's sarcoma is encountered, frequently invading the gastro-intestinal tract and various internal organs, causing severe disease and death (Fig. 1.4). Another tumour characteristic of AIDS is lymphoma, a malignancy of lymphoid tissue in the lymph glands and also in various organs of the body, for example the spleen, bone marrow and liver. The cellular elements of the immune system constitute to a large extent the lymphoid system of the body together with connective tissue and connective tissue cells. Malignancy of these cells, termed lymphoma or lymphatic leukaemia (if it is predominantly in the blood), is frequently associated with viral infections. In the lymphomas associated with AIDS, the Epstein–Barr virus, also a member of the herpes family, has been incriminated as having a role in the development of this malignancy. Another disease associated with Epstein–Barr virus infection in AIDS patients is a lesion found in the mouth and usually also on the tongue called oral hairy leukoplakia (leukos = white; plakia = plaque), which consists of white patches with a roughened 'hairy' appearance. These lesions may go on to develop into malignancy at a later stage.

The clinical stages of HIV infection

HIV infection had, until relatively recently, been portrayed as a typical example of a slow virus disease of Man. The term 'slow' virus disease refers to the prolonged course of the infection following a lengthy incubation period (that is, the time from infection until the clinical manifestations of disease). The clinical course of the disease does indeed resemble that of other slow virus diseases. Following infection with a virus which may produce clinical symptoms referred to as the acute HIV syndrome, there is a long, silent phase lasting from eight to 15 years. During this phase there are no symptoms and the patient outwardly appears to be quite healthy. Furthermore, the virus is at a low level in the blood and is detectable only with very sensitive techniques such as the polymerase chain reaction (PCR) discussed in Chapter 5. Laboratory tests for immune function or assays which count the number of CD4 lymphocytes in the blood show little or no disturbances of function or depletion in cell numbers, unlike the profound changes seen in the more advanced stages of the disease. Generally speaking, it is only the antibodies in the blood which indicate that the patient is, in fact, infected. However, this clinical calmness deceptively conceals the titanic struggle which takes place in the patient's body between rapidly replicating HIV and the frantic attempts of the CD4 population to replenish the vast number of cells destroyed by the virus. Studies of HIV-infected patients demonstrated that in the clinically 'silent' phase of infection some 100 million virus particles are produced and destroyed daily while, at the same time, about 2000 million CD4 lymphocytes, or 5% of the total population, are destroyed by the virus every day and need to be replaced by regeneration of cells. These findings illustrate the truly remarkable capacity of the body's immune system to be able to resist this immense viral onslaught. It has also been shown that the main mass of the virus resides not in the bloodstream but in the lymphoid tissue of the body and it is here, rather than in the bloodstream, where the contest between virus and lymphocyte occurs in the main. Not surprisingly, therefore, the level of virus in the bloodstream is low or barely detectable during the clinically silent phase of the illness.

For a number of years the body is able to replace the CD4 lymphocytes that are destroyed by the virus. Eventually, however, the immune system becomes exhausted and there is a progressive destruction of the architecture of the lymphoid tissue. Replenishment of CD4 lymphocytes fails to keep up with the destruction by the virus, resulting in a sharp increase in the amount of virus and a corresponding precipitous drop in the number of CD4 lymphocytes in the bloodstream, ultimately resulting in a profound depression of immune function.

Usually the first clinical sign to be manifest is enlargement and swelling of the lymph nodes, called lymphadenopathy, seen especially in the head and neck region. This clinical stage is referred to as progressive generalized lymphadenopathy (PGL) or the lymphadenopathy syndrome (LAS). However, swelling of the lymph nodes is, in itself, not an uncommon clinical finding and many other viruses, for example the glandular fever virus (Epstein–Barr), CMV and other organisms, can also produce this. It is therefore not specific for HIV infection and this clinical syndrome, on its own, is not a diagnostic criterion for the disease of AIDS.

At a somewhat later stage, further clinical signs of HIV infection may become evident including weight loss, diarrhoea, fever and recurrent thrush infections of the oral and genital mucous membranes. These symptoms now do become highly suggestive of AIDS, but again are not necessarily specific and diagnostic of AIDS, and this stage is often referred to as pre-AIDS or AIDS-related complex (ARC).

The exact clinical criteria to diagnose the stage of AIDS itself have undergone a number of changes over the years and a dozen or so different AIDS classifications have been proposed by various organizations such as the Centers for Disease Control (CDC) and WHO. Different sets of criteria have also been suggested for Africa because of the difference in the spectrum of opportunistic infections and the lack of adequate diagnostic capabilities for laboratory testing for HIV infection, immune function and many of the opportunistic infections. The stage of AIDS itself is eventually diagnosed when the minimal clinical criteria, depending on the classification system used, become manifest in the patient.

There are therefore four clinical stages of HIV infections – the acute HIV syndrome, the silent (latent) stage, PGL, ARC and AIDS itself.

Acute HIV syndrome

This syndrome is also referred to as 'seroconversion illness' as it coincides with the individual converting from having no antibodies in the serum, to becoming positive for HIV antibodies. The illness occurs some two to four weeks after infection and lasts about one to two weeks, after which the patient recovers and is henceforth seropositive for HIV antibodies. Typically, the illness is sudden in onset and characterized by a fever, swelling of the lymph glands, a measles-like rash over the whole body and ulcers in the mouth and sometimes genitalia. Many of these features resemble glandular fever (also called infectious mononucleosis) and the syndrome used to be referred to as 'mononucleosis-like'. There are, however, now recognized to be clear distinctions between these two illnesses. Disease of the gastro-intestinal tract is often involved, manifesting as anorexia, nausea, vomiting and diarrhoea. In the mouth, in addition to the ulcers in the mucous membrane, there is often inflammation of the pharynx and there may be pain on swallowing. Not infrequently the nervous system is affected and there may be a meningitis (inflammation of the meninges, the covering of the brain) or an encephalitis (inflammation of brain tissue itself), with a spectrum of neurological signs. Fatigue, lethargy and depression are characteristic of the illness and may persist for weeks to months after recovery.

At the early stage there may well be a profound suppression of the immune system seen on laboratory testing, but also manifest by severe opportunistic infections, especially thrush. At this early stage in the course of infection there is a large amount of virus in the bloodstream which is quite readily detectable by laboratory testing.

The acute HIV syndrome by no means occurs in all individuals infected with the virus and many individuals who are HIV positive do not recall ever having experienced the illness. Estimates vary as to how frequently it does occur, the commonly accepted rate being 50% to 70%. This range would naturally be higher in individuals who would be particularly on the look-out for it after being knowingly exposed to HIV. Of interest, the acute HIV syndrome is rarely seen in children.

The silent phase

During this stage of the natural history of HIV, the individual is not aware clinically of being infected. Laboratory tests such as the antibody test are positive, but the presence of virus is usually not as readily detectable at this stage as during the acute illness. Nevertheless, individuals are still undoubtedly infectious (i.e. are capable of transmitting infection) during the silent phase. After the acute illness immune function returns to normal and on laboratory testing an HIV-infected individual may well have a totally normal immune profile. However, as time goes on, and as the viral load increases in the body involving more and more of the immune system, signs of immunological suppression start appearing and becoming progressively worse. Laboratory tests for immune function may reveal very marked immunosuppression before the onset of opportunistic infections. Sooner or later clinical signs and symptoms develop and the patient then advances to the next stage, that of the progressive generalized lymphadenopathy.

Progressive generalized lymphadenopathy (PGL)

During this stage the patient becomes aware that the lymph glands, especially in the head and neck region, are swollen and are easily felt under the skin. In some cases they become so enlarged that they are visible and the patient may become aware of them looking in the mirror, or may see or feel them while shaving. These lymph glands may fluctuate and decrease or increase in size, but generally the enlargement persists for long periods of time and is an important clinical sign of HIV infection. The status of the immune system is unrelated to the presence or absence of PGL. The stage of PGL is by no means invariable and many HIV-infected individuals may bypass it and go straight from the silent stage to the established AIDS stage.

The AIDS-related complex (ARC)

The concept of a discrete stage of ARC is one that is not universally accepted by all clinicians. As the name suggests, ARC is a composite of clinical symptoms and signs which precede the advent of AIDS itself. The composite is, however, not diagnostic of AIDS, although, as with PGL, it is an important diagnostic stage of HIV infection. Many clinicians who do not accept the concept of ARC feel that the signs and symptoms comprising ARC should rather be incorporated into the definition of AIDS itself, and indeed a number of classification systems do just that. In either event, the immune system does, at this stage, show laboratory signs of very significant, if not profound, immunosuppression.

The components of the ARC complex have been alluded to above and consist essentially of the three non-specific presentations of chronic pyrexia, chronic diarrhoea and weight loss, together with some opportunistic infections that are not specific indicator diseases of AIDS, such as thrush.

AIDS

The diagnostic elements of this end-stage of HIV infection have undergone various changes under different classification systems over the years. The advent of AIDS marks an important milestone in the course of the infection. An irreversible step has been reached when the diagnosis of AIDS is made. Recovery from individual opportunistic infections may well occur and there may also be remission from the tumours. However they do recur, usually with increasing severity and frequency and become more and more difficult to treat until finally the patient dies, on average after about 18 months to two years after the onset of disease.

Essentially the components of AIDS consist of the direct consequences of damage by HIV as well as the indirect consequences of immunosuppression. The direct effects involve various organs, for example the central nervous system (CNS), the gut, the blood-forming elements, the kidneys, joints and skin. There are also direct general effects on the body comprising the three elements of ARC, which in AIDS patients become more severe often with very profound wasting, as well as the very characteristic skeletal-like picture of AIDS patients. Commonly, premature greying of hair and wrinkling of skin occur, rapidly ageing the patient's appearance.

The clinical presentation of the opportunistic infections depends on which organism is responsible and which organs are infected. Also the tumour presentations will depend on the type of tumour and the site or sites of the body that are affected.

AIDS classification systems

A number of different classification systems have been introduced by various international agencies and other bodies. The first classification system, introduced in 1982 by the CDC, established a set of clinical criteria necessary for the diagnosis of AIDS. The purpose of this classification system was to enable field workers to carry out surveillance of the number of individuals affected and to monitor the progress of the disease. In the field, various surveillance definitions have been assessed for sensitivity; that is, whether they are sufficiently broad to be able to pick up as many individuals with AIDS as possible, including those who may not have many of the prescribed criteria. They were also assessed for specificity; that is, whether the criteria were sufficiently restrictive so as not to include too many other clinical conditions which could give similar signs and symptoms. As a result of ongoing evaluations, the classification systems for AIDS have been modified and amended from time to time as more and more is learnt about the disease. With the advent of laboratory tests for HIV infection, the presence of detectable HIV antibodies was incorporated as a diagnostic criterion, together with laboratory evidence of immunosuppression. Since 1982, several CDC classification systems have been published in addition to those from other bodies.

Essentially the classification systems for AIDS consist of three major features: firstly, laboratory tests for HIV infection as well as for immunosuppression; secondly, demonstration of what are called indicator diseases, that is the specific opportunistic infections or tumours which predict that the individual is at least significantly immunosuppressed; thirdly, the cerebral manifestations of AIDS as well as the other direct effects of the virus such as wasting. Classification systems have been modified for specific circumstances; for example, in 1986 the WHO at a meeting in Bangui, in the Central African Republic, proposed a working definition for Africa which soon became known as the Bangui definition. This classification was tailored for African conditions where the spectrum of opportunistic infections is different from that in the USA and Europe, and it also makes provisions for the inadequacies in laboratory testing facilities in many African countries, both for HIV as well as for a number of the opportunistic infections. A specific classification system for children was established by the CDC in 1987 and has also, since then, undergone some modifications.

In addition to standards for the diagnosis of AIDS a number of classification systems for the staging of HIV disease have been published. In practice many clinicians utilize the broad divisions of the acute phase, the silent phase, PGL, ARC and AIDS. However, more exact prognostic staging systems have been established by various bodies. One of the earliest of these, the Walter Reed system of 1986, so-called after the Walter Reed Hospital where it was initially devised, makes use of the clinical presentation as well as laboratory tests for the extent of immune dysfunction. A more recent WHO/CDC staging system was published in 1990 and couples clinical criteria to scales of performance. There are four clinical stages ranging from asymptomatic infection to established AIDS (stage 4), the performance scale in the latter representing an individual bedridden for over half of the day during the previous month.

HIV and the CNS

Infection of the CNS by HIV results in a wide range of clinical presentations. The disease manifestations and syndromes of the CNS are among the most complex clinical aspects of AIDS. As mentioned previously, nervous tissue is one of the two major targets for HIV. Infection of the brain and the immune system proceed in parallel. Thus, while damage to the immune system produces the clinical presentations detailed above, at the same time infection and damage to the CNS together result in their own spectrum of disease presentations. Neurological involvement may therefore occur during any of the stages of HIV infection. Also, the CNS may be involved as a result of direct damage by HIV or as a result of opportunistic infections or tumours which can, and often do, cause CNS disease.

The CNS in the acute HIV syndrome

Acute meningitis or encephalitis may, as we have seen, be a component of the acute HIV syndrome. Other acute manifestations may also occur, such as acute neuritis (inflammation of a single nerve), or polyneuritis (inflammation of many peripheral nerves of the body).

The CNS in the silent phase

By definition the silent phase is characterized by the absence of any clinical signs or symptoms of infection, but is only evident on laboratory testing. So too, in the case of CNS – by definition there ought not to be any clinically overt signs of infection. However, a number of studies carried out since 1986 on asymptomatically infected individuals have initiated a major storm of controversy which has still not yet been resolved. Using psychometric testing procedures to measure the functional ability of infected individuals to perform mental tasks, research workers are able to demonstrate established deficiencies in asymptomatically infected individuals. These deficiencies ranged from impaired cognition (that is the ability to understand), slowing down of reasoning ability, memory difficulties, decreased problem-solving abilities and reduced fine motor co-ordination. Coupled with the neurophysiological deficits, a variety of psychiatric disorders were also diagnosed in these individuals.

The demonstration of these neurophysiological and neuropsychiatric disorders in ostensibly asymptomatically infected individuals created a critical question mark over the abilities of HIV-infected individuals to function satisfactorily and safely in sensitive work situations. For example, taking charge of heavy machinery, driving buses and trains or flying aircraft. It also raised the issue of the need for compulsory HIV testing of individuals aspiring to be trained or to be employed in vocations where public safety could be endangered. The WHO was, however, swift to refute the implications of these studies and in early 1988 published an assurance that, in its view, and on the weight of existing scientific knowledge, there was no evidence that otherwise healthy HIV-infected individuals were any more functionally impaired than uninfected persons. Certainly, other than through detailed psychometric testing or psychiatric evaluation, no signs of CNS involvement are usually detectable in the majority of asymptomatically infected persons. This is unlike the situation in the symptomatic stages of HIV infection, where physical signs of cerebral damage and destruction of brain tissue due to depletion of neurones (brain cells) are frequently seen on brain scan and EEG (EEG = encephalogram, a recording of the brain's electrical activity), and neurophysiological and neuropsychiatric disturbances are always detectable. It is also very difficult to distinguish reactive changes and deficiencies in mental functioning (and also psychiatric difficulties which are the result of an individual being confronted with a profound diagnosis of HIV with all its implications) from organic disease due to HIV infection of the brain. A further meeting of the WHO held early in 1990 again confirmed that there was no scientific evidence of mental functional deficiency in asymptomatically infected individuals. However, the disquiet over the issue has still not been settled. A multicultural study in six centres in the USA, Europe, the Far East and Africa was established by the WHO in 1991 to try and obtain further clarification on this important issue.

CNS disease due to direct HIV viral damage

There are three main clinical results of infection of the nervous system by HIV and the consequent damage to nervous tissue in established HIV infection: HIV encephalopathy (damage to the brain), HIV myelopathy (damage to the spinal cord) and peripheral neuropathy (damage to the peripheral nerves of the body).

The term encephalopathy denotes damage to the brain. Sometimes the more specific term HIV encephalitis, to denote inflammation of the brain, is used. (The older term subacute encephalitis is no longer in common usage.) AIDS dementia complex refers to the clinical presentation in the later stages of HIV encephalopathy. Because the targeting of nervous tissue for infection by HIV is a functional property of the virus, it is assumed to occur invariably, irrespective of whether it is clinically manifest or not. Infection results in destruction and loss of neurones which cannot be replenished. There follows a progressive diminution and contraction of the brain which is quite clearly seen on brain scan (Fig. 1.5). The earlier clinical stages of HIV encephalopathy seen as subtle neurophysiological deficiencies (which may or may not occur in the silent phase of the disease) are invariably seen in established AIDS disease. During the more advanced stages of HIV encephalopathy, more gross clinical signs of AIDS dementia may occur which may then become the dominant clinical presentation of AIDS, and ultimately be the cause of death. The earliest signs of dementia are those of functional deficiencies in mental ability followed by loss of memory, confusion, disorientation, hallucinations and eventually psychotic behaviour. Occasionally there may also be neurological signs such as aphasia (central disturbance of speech function), ataxia (disturbance of gait), paralysis and others. In the late stages the patient may lapse into stupor and coma before death.

Involvement of the spinal cord – HIV myelopathy, also called vacuolar myelopathy (to describe the typical microscopical pathological al cord tissue consisting of large balloon-like 'holes' or vacuoles) – occurs only in the established stage of AIDS. Destruction of spinal cord nervous tissue results in paralysis of the lower limbs, frequently together with urinary and faecal incontinence and impotence.

Damage to the peripheral nerves may diffusely involve many peripheral nerves and presents clinically as a feeling of pins and needles in the early stages due to irritation of the nerves, but at a later stage may become very painful and still later, with destruction of nervous tissue, can result in loss of sensation to the affected parts of the body or paralysis of the relevant muscles. Occasionally single nerves may be involved which is referred to as mononeuritis. For example, involvement of the facial nerve may produce a paralysis of the muscles on one side of the face called Bell's palsy.

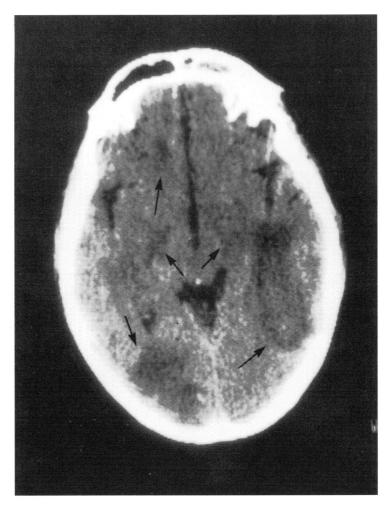

Fig. 1.5 Brain scan of patient with AIDS dementia, showing multiple areas of low density (indicated by arrows), consistent with brain atrophy. (Photograph courtesy of Dr D C Spencer.)

CNS disease due to opportunistic infections and tumours

The brain, as with many other organs, may be involved in the opportunistic infections of AIDS and virtually all of the organisms mentioned earlier can infect the brain, the notable exception being *Pneumocystis carinii*, which appears to be virtually confined to the lung. Similarly, the tumours characteristic of AIDS, the lymphomas and Kaposi's sarcoma, may also spread to the brain causing CNS disease.

AIDS in children

This generally follows the same pattern as seen in adults, although the incubation period is considerably shorter and the course of the disease more rapid. The majority of children are infected at or soon after birth from an infected mother or following blood transfusion. The disease is then silent and may, in the early stages, be difficult to diagnose, even by laboratory testing, because antibodies may have diffused from the mother's bloodstream into that of the infant and maternal antibodies may still be present in the infant's bloodstream for up to 15 months without the infant necessarily having been actively infected.

The spectrum of disease is somewhat different from that in adults; some of the opportunistic infections of adults are rare in children, for example toxoplasmosis and cryptococcus infections. The tumours seen in adults, Kaposi's sarcoma and lymphoma, are also uncommon in children. However, malignant proliferation of lymphocytes – called lymphocytic infiltrative disease which may involve many organs, especially the lungs in which it causes pneumonia – is far more common in children than in adults. The classification system developed specifically for children by the CDC in 1987 takes these differences into account in its formulation of diagnostic criteria for paediatric AIDS.

The prognosis and course of HIV disease

Possibly one of the most agonizing questions in the counselling of HIV-positive individuals relates to the long-term prognosis of the infection. How many HIV-infected individuals will go on to develop AIDS? How soon after infection does AIDS occur? Once the disease of AIDS has occurred, what is the outlook?

Many studies have been carried out on groups of infected individuals and AIDS patients to try and answer these questions. Results from early follow-up studies of HIV-infected individuals suggested that only a minority of infected persons would go on to develop AIDS – anything from 10% to 30%. However, as these follow-up studies were extended for longer periods of time it became apparent that these figures were overly optimistic. The majority of follow-up studies have been carried out on groups of homosexual men in Western countries which generally have high standards of medical care and these individuals are usually well motivated and often health-conscious. Thus, figures coming from these studies probably reflect a somewhat more favourable prognostic viewpoint. The rates of progression from HIV infection to AIDS have been reported as 0–2% after two years, 5–10% after four years, 10–25% after six years, 30–40% after eight years and about 50% after ten years.

An important group of HIV-infected individuals are the so-called long-term non-progressors. These are people known to be infected with HIV for seven or more years, but with no symptoms of disease and retaining a good immune function with no evidence of significant depletion of their CD4 lymphocytes despite not having received any antiviral therapy. It would appear that these individuals have a particularly robust immune system, able to effectively suppress HIV replication and halt the progression of the course of infection. Research institutions throughout the world have been intensively studying these individuals in an effort to understand which aspects of the immune system are of particular importance in controlling HIV infection. How long these patients are able to stave off progression of disease or, indeed, whether there are some who may permanently escape AIDS is still not known.

Recent advances in antiviral therapy (Chapter 6) have now reached a stage where sustained interruption in the progression of disease can be achieved, if therapy is commenced at a relatively early stage in the course of infection. There are a number of authorities who now believe that HIV may, in fact, now be a curable infection if optimal antiretroviral therapy is started early enough after infection. It has, in fact, even been computed that if optimal antiviral therapy is able to maintain the reduction of the amount of virus in the blood to undetectable levels, the infection could be eradicated within a time period of between 2.3 and 3.1 years. (This is not an opinion shared by most authorities.) It has not been satisfactorily answered as yet whether all HIV-infected individuals eventually develop AIDS.

In untreated patients the rate of progression depends on a number of factors including the stage of infection, age, socio-economic factors and ethnicity. In the early stages of infection, relatively few cases of HIV infection progress to AIDS. As time wears on a higher and higher percentage convert to AIDS. The average time from initial infection to AIDS for an adult is estimated at about 8–13 years for HIV-1 and 10–15 years for HIV-2. Few studies have been carried out on other at-risk groups, for example intravenous drug abusers, and similarly little is known as yet about the rate of progression in African patients where the prognosis appears to be considerably worse. In children the course of the disease is also much more rapid. The average incubation period for children is less than five years and, where children have been infected in infancy as is usually the case, the average incubation period can be as short as two years.

The prognosis for established AIDS disease itself is bleak. At our present state of knowledge, recovery from AIDS is not known to occur and the disease is always fatal. The average survival time for AIDS due to HIV-1 is 18 months to two years, with that due to HIV-2 being somewhat longer. There have, however, now been recorded a number of cases of AIDS patients who have survived for as long as 10 years after the onset of disease. Undoubtedly factors such as the level of health care and early diagnosis of opportunistic infections, antiviral therapy, state of physical and mental health at the time of infection, motivation and state of mind regarding the infection, absence of continuing exposure to the virus and limitation of exposure to potential opportunistic infections are all significant factors that can improve the prognosis of the individual both in terms of progression to AIDS as well as the course of AIDS itself.

Clearly, the cardinal feature of HIV infection and its subsequent diseases is its inexorable progression in the majority of cases. Also, once an individual is infected, he or she remains infectious, that is he or she is able to transmit the infection to others, for a lifetime. Finally, as we have seen, most infected persons eventually get HIV related diseases and established AIDS is still universally fatal. All of these aspects taken together make HIV a unique infection in humans and AIDS a unique disease.

2

The AIDS virus

Before examining the features of the AIDS virus it may be as well to look first at some of the characteristics of viruses in general, for there are few biological concepts that have become so much a part of common parlance and that are so misunderstood.

What is a virus?

The word 'virus' is derived from the Latin word meaning 'poison' and also 'slimy material'. It is still defined in most English dictionaries as a malignant or morbid poison. In medical circles the word 'virus' often overlaps with the word 'germ' in a vague and diffuse way to connote some infectious organism which can make do for the diagnosis of a patient's ills where no other apparent cause is forthcoming. (The patient is also further reassured that the 'virus is going around anyway'.) The word 'virus' has now even been taken over by the computer world to denote an infectious corruption of data banks which is transmissible between computers in epidemic and even pandemic fashion.

In the biological world, however, viruses are definite entities and although only recognized and described within scientific parameters since the end of the last century, have been intensively studied and characterized down to molecular and even atomic levels. Yet few scientists would venture to define in a single short sentence what a virus is. Rather, it is easier to describe a virus by its characteristics and properties when viewed from a structural, functional or clinical point of view.

A structural definition of a virus

As a structural entity the virus represents the simplest biological unit able to exist and to perpetuate itself by making copies of itself (replication). Its simplicity is reflected in the frequently used description of viruses being on the 'threshold of life'. In common with higher forms of life a virus needs genes in order to make copies of itself. Genes form the master code which houses the blueprint for the design of the organism, that is what the organism consists of and how it functions. The message for the blueprint is written into the sequence in which the building blocks (which consist of molecules called nucleotides) are strung together in a highly specific order to form a long chain called nucleic acid. The sum total of the genes of an organism, viruses or higher forms of life, is called the genome of that organism. As mentioned in the Introduction, the genome of higher organisms is always DNA (deoxyribose nucleic acid – the nucleic acid type where the linker molecule is a deoxyribose sugar), whereas in viruses it may be DNA or RNA (ribonucleic acid – the nucleic acid type where the sugar linker molecule is ribose).

The second structural component that a virus needs is a shell to surround and protect the nucleic acid genome and also to act as a vehicle to convey the virus from cell to cell and also from organism to organism. The shell, which in scientific terms is referred to as a capsid, is composed of protein building blocks assembled in a crystalline structure to give the virus strength; it also imparts to the virus a characteristic appearance by which it is recognizable under the electron microscope. On the outside of the shell are specific proteins which allow the virus to recognize binding sites (also called receptor sites) on the surface of cells that it will infect. In addition to the capsid, many but not all viruses have a third component, an envelope, which is a loose, fragile membrane covering the capsid and derived partly from the cell membrane of the host cell.

A functional definition of a virus

Given the extreme structural simplicity of viruses and the fact that they consist of the barest minimum requirements of living forms, viruses have no capacity to generate their own energy requirements for various biochemical processes such as replication. They also lack the machinery to enable them to synthesize their own proteins and nucleic acids. To carry out these extra biological processes, viruses need to make use of the host cell's machinery and biochemical facilities, which may or may not be to the detriment of the cell. The virus, therefore, is dependent on infecting a living cell in order for it to be able to replicate itself. In fact, outside of a living cell, a virus is nothing more than a group of inert chemicals; it is only 'alive' inside host cells. Therefore, while most higher micro-organisms are able to live on inert organic media, viruses are all, by definition, obligate intra-cellular parasites. The purloining of the cell's resources and facilities for use by the virus may or may not result in obvious damage to the cell; that is, a virus may or may not be pathogenic (able to produce disease) to the cell.

A genetic definition of a virus

A molecular geneticist (a scientist who studies the genetics of organisms at a molecular level) may view a virus as a biological entity that transmits genetic information between cells. The virus, being an obligate intracellular parasite and, by definition, being infectious, transports its own genetic material between the cells that it infects and also between the individuals that it infects. In doing so it may leave behind some of its nucleic acid which could be integrated, and eventually even incorporated, into the genetic constitution of the new host. Viruses may also pick up genetic material from the host's genome or from other viruses which may happen to be in the cell at the same time and then incorporate this extraneous nucleic acid into its own genome. In this way viruses may act as dissemi-nators of genetic material between organisms in much the same way as bees spread pollen from plant to plant. Viruses may well be a significant factor in promoting genetic diversity in animal species and in this way play a role, in addition to causing mutation, in the genetic changes which favour evolutionary adaptation.

A clinical definition of a virus

A clinical definition would describe a virus as a transmissible micro-organism responsible for a wide variety of human diseases with clinical presentations characteristic for each of the different viruses. A further feature of the clinical definition of viruses is their resistance to antibiotics which differentiates them from higher microbiological forms of life, such as bacteria. This resistance is also a consequence of the simplicity of the virus, which has few biochemical pathways of its own and therefore affords little in the way of targets for antibiotics or antimicrobial drugs to act on.

The size of viruses

As well as being the simplest, viruses are also the smallest of living agents. The unit of measurement used for viruses is the nanometer (or nm) – 1 nm is a thousandth of a micrometer (µm), the unit of measurement used for

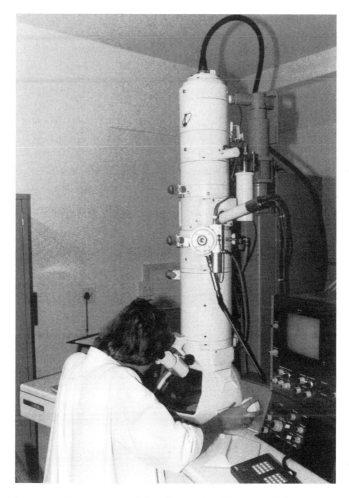

Fig. 2.1 Electron microscope used for direct visualization of viruses.

micro-organisms such as bacteria, and the micrometer is, in turn, a thousandth of a millimeter (mm). In other words, one nanometer is equal to a millionth of a millimeter. Viruses vary in size from about 22 nm in diameter through to the largest and most complex of the viruses, the pox virus, which has dimensions of about 200–400 nm. The smallest object visible in the light microscope is just at the limit of the pox viruses in size, and these viruses may be barely visible under the light microscope. The vast majority of viruses, however, can be visualized only using the electron microscope – an instrument that utilizes electrons beamed from a high-tension electron gun into a very high vacuum (Fig. 2.1). The beam is magnified, after it has passed through the virus, by a series of magnetic fields, and is then visualized on a fluorescent screen which glows when the electrons come into contact with it.

The structure of viruses

As viruses vary widely in their sizes, so too do they correspondingly vary in their complexity. The smallest and simplest of viruses may have only some three to four genes and the protein building blocks made by a single gene are repetitively run off the same gene and then assembled to form the capsid. The largest and most complex of the viruses may have a few hundred genes including a sizeable number of its own enzymes. The genome of viruses, either RNA or DNA, may be in the form of a single long strand or it may be chopped up into fragments, usually each fragment representing a single gene. It may consist of a single strand of nucleic acid or it may be double-stranded, as is the case in higher forms of life, with a sequence on the one strand being a mirror image of its complementary strand. The length of a genome is often expressed in terms of the number of nucleotide building blocks (or bases as they are also commonly referred to). Thus, a small virus may have a genome of only 3000 bases (or 3 kilo- bases – 3 kb) with the most complex being several hundred kilobases in length. A gene is generally of the order of 1 kb in length. However, in many situations, there may be a sharing of nucleotide sequences between genes; that is, the full sequence of one gene may overlap with part of the sequence of another. Thus the total number of genes may well be more than the number suggested by the length of the nucleic acid.

The capsid of the virus is constructed in one of three ways. The protein building blocks may be strung out like a necklace, which is then wound spirally to form a tightly coiled spring. This type of capsid is called a heli- cal capsid. A second type of capsid structure commonly found in viruses is formed by protein building blocks which are assembled into a cubical crystalline structure. In the large pox viruses the type of capsid found here is called a complex capsid.

The third structure seen in many viruses is the envelope which the virus derives partly by budding through the cell membrane. Viral proteins are encrusted into the inner surface of the envelope but, more importantly, they are also found in the form of spikes embedded into the outer surface of the envelope and protruding to the outside of the virus. These spikes play an important role in attaching the virus to its specific receptors on the host cell.

Classification of viruses

On the basis of these structural features, viruses may be classified into various groups. Thus, the two broad groups of viruses are the RNA viruses and the DNA viruses. They can then also be subdivided on the basis of the genome of the virus into double-stranded or single-stranded and fragmented or single chained. Also, the presence or absence of an envelope is an important classification criterion; that is, viruses are broadly divided into two groups – enveloped or non-enveloped viruses. Finally the shape and size of the capsid is also used for classification.

The broadest grouping of viruses is the family. Viruses which share a few basic characteristics, such as being either DNA or RNA, enveloped or non-enveloped, cubical or helical and approximately the same size, could belong to the same family. Within families, viruses are further grouped together on the basis of closer similarities in size of genome, finer structural details and protein or other biochemical similarities. These groups are called genera (singular = genus), and within genera are species. It should be emphasized that these groupings are based on virological features and not on the kinds of diseases they produce. There are very commonly instances of viruses that are closely related to each other and are classified within the same family but cause completely different diseases and are spread in markedly different ways. For example, the virus causing the common childhood illness of rubella (german measles) is virologically related to the insect-borne viruses called arboviruses which are clinically and epidemiologically markedly different. Conversely there are frequent situations where similar clinical diseases are caused by viruses that biologically are radically different from each other, for example the five completely separate viruses that cause viral hepatitis.

The isolation and growth of viruses

The isolation of viruses from human specimens and their propagation for further study is something which often intrigues non-virologists. Viruses are obligate intracellular parasites; that is, they cannot exist without a host and therefore they cannot be isolated or grown in the same way as other micro-organisms (e.g. bacteria), on liquid or solid nutritive media in plates or in flasks. In order to grow viruses a supply of living cells is needed. These can be in the form of living animals and, in the early stages of virology, inoculation of laboratory animals was the only way of isolating and growing viruses. In the modern virology laboratory, infant mice (usually within 24 hours of birth) are sometimes used to isolate certain viruses. The

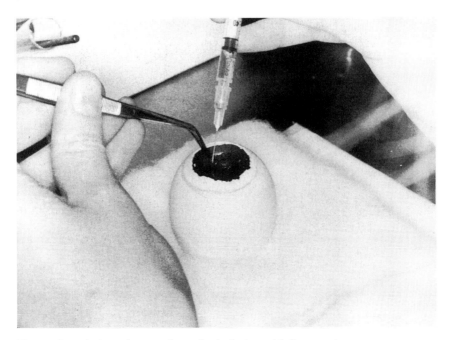

Fig 2.2 Inoculation of egg embryo for isolation of influenza virus.

embryos of fertilized chicken eggs are regularly used for isolation of viruses such as influenza (Fig. 2.2) and also for the large-scale growth of influenza and yellow fever viruses for the manufacture of vaccines.

In the main, however, it is cell cultures that are used for the isolation and propagation of most viruses. Cells that are obtained from animal organs or from aborted human foetuses are suspended in a nutritive medium and attach to and grow on the surface of plastic or glass flasks (Fig. 2.3). With some kinds of cells, the culture remains in suspension rather than adhering to a surface. For vaccine production, where large masses of cultured cells are required, vast fermentation vats of cell cultures are usually used, where temperature, oxygenation and media conditions are computer controlled. In diagnostic laboratories cell cultures are put into small test tubes or even into small depressions in plastic plates to be incubated with human material for the isolation of viruses (Fig. 2.4). The presence of viruses in these cultures can then be identified in various ways. Some viruses produce morphological changes in the cells which can be recognized under the microscope. In other cases more indirect techniques are used to detect viral growth; for example, techniques to demonstrate the presence of viral proteins in the cells or in the media. In the diagnostic

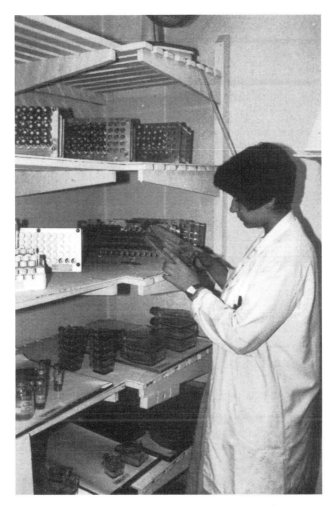

Fig. 2.3 Incubator room for large-scale propagation of cell cultures.

laboratory it is often inconvenient to have to depend on cell cultures derived
from animal organs or foetuses; instead, continuous cell cultures, which
can be propagated over and over again without dying off, are frequently
used. These continuous cultures, which are also called line cells, are usually
derived from cancerous tissue and are therefore not used to make vaccines.

In the modern diagnostic virology laboratory techniques other than
isolation are frequently used to detect the presence of viruses, and indeed
a number of important human viruses cannot be grown in culture at all
or only with great difficulty, and these alternative techniques are needed

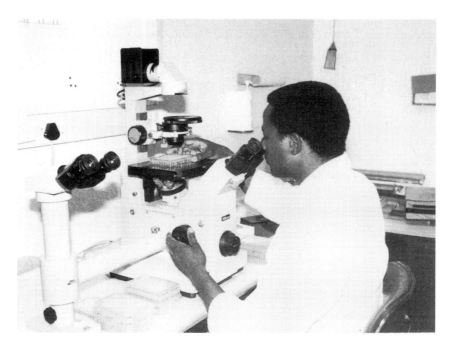

Fig 2.4 Plastic microtite plates inoculated with material from patients being examined for the presence of viruses

for their detection. These include techniques to demonstrate the protein components of the virus by serological techniques or the demonstration of viral nucleic acid. The principle of these tests will be discussed more fully in Chapter 5.

How do viruses cause disease?

Many viruses replicate in cells without causing any apparent damage or disturbance to the cell. Others may cause some subtle functional disturbances, especially to highly specialized cells such as neurones, without killing them or causing any structural damage. However, many virus infections are lethal to the host cell, in some cases slowly over a number of days or even weeks, whereas with virulent viruses cells may be killed within 12 hours of infection.

There are a number of mechanisms by which viral replication inside cells can cause damage and death of the cell. An obvious one is the diversion of resources including materials, energy and manufacturing facilities away from the cell to the virus. Accumulation of virus particles inside the cell can also physically damage the cell by osmosis; that is, the drawing of water into the cell thus increasing the hydrostatic pressure inside it. Virus replication may physically damage or puncture delicate membranes inside the cell. There are also a number of biochemical ways in which viruses can damage cells. Some viral capsid proteins are directly toxic to cells and production and accumulation of these proteins can themselves cause cell damage and death. A number of viruses also produce soluble proteins to specifically switch off the cell's metabolic processes and actively divert resources to the virus. These viral protein 'messengers' may pass a signal to damage and even kill the cell. Another mechanism that relates to a number of viruses, especially enveloped viruses, is the fusing of membranes of cells to each other to produce giant cells, also called syncytia. This fusion process is an extension of the early step of replication of enveloped viruses, which need to fuse their envelopes with the cell membrane in order for the virus to gain entry into the cell for replication. The virus protein, which causes this fusion process, can thus also cause cell membranes to fuse to each other and result in syncytia which are cells that are profoundly damaged and not able to survive for long. Finally, viruses may initiate a sequence of biochemical changes which ultimately lead to the death of the cell. This programmed cell death, which can also be set in motion by a variety of other triggers, is called apoptosis and is thought to be an important mechanism by which many viruses, including HIV, kill cells.

All these mechanisms of cell damage and death operate in cultured cells infected with viruses. In the intact body, however, there are additional indirect mechanisms for cell damage and death. When viruses infect and replicate inside cells their proteins are often found on the surface of the cell. These viral proteins are not recognized as belonging to the protein make-up of that individual and are perceived by the immune surveillance system as 'foreign', and this then sets up an immune response to attempt to rid the body of this intruding foreign protein material. The consequent inflammatory and immune responses directed against the infected cell often themselves cause damage to the cell containing the virus as well as to uninfected neighbouring cells and thus the inflammatory response itself contributes to the disease process. Other indirect mechanisms that may operate include infection of cells in the blood vessels which may cause obstruction, thus shutting off the blood supply to tissues, with consequent pathology or damage to blood vessels, which may result in haemorrhage or loss of fluid into surrounding tissue.

The disease consequences of the destruction of cells are as much a result of the extent of the damage as which particular cells are damaged. Clearly subtle damage to highly sensitive and critical cells, for example in the central nervous system, will cause a greater severity of disease than even extensive cellular damage in an organ which is large and can regenerate tissue easily, for example the gastro-intestinal tract, liver or muscle. To some extent the subjective expression of disease is also dependent on the milieu in which the infection occurs; for example, the threshold for feelings of ill-health are quite markedly different in street urchins in Africa than they would be in pampered socialites in New York City.

Thus, to get a clearer idea of the terminology which is used one needs to examine carefully the meaning of the words 'infection' and 'disease'. 'Infection' merely denotes that a micro-organism is established and multiplying in the body. 'Disease' denotes the consequent malfunctioning of the body, which can be demonstrated by tests for organ functions or by clinical examination, or by subjective feelings of ill-health.

The range of diseases caused by viruses

As discussed above, a wide spectrum of effects may result from viral infections of cells, ranging from no effect to rapid death. Virulent viruses such as poliomyelitis or herpes simplex virus can cause death of cells within hours of infection. Such infections are termed acute cytocidal effects (cyto- = cell, -cidal = killing). At the other end of the spectrum there are many examples of viruses living and multiplying harmoniously together with the host cell. Such infections are termed latent or non-cytocidal infections and are seen characteristically in members of the herpes virus family. The latent stage may persist for a lifetime or the virus–cell relationship may be changed by triggering factors that can activate the virus to start multiplying at a much higher rate ultimately causing cell damage and death. An extreme form of latency is found in the case of viral genes which are permanently integrated into the chromosome of the host cell. Thus, the only way in which these viruses can even be detected is by a diligent search for the presence of the particular gene or genes within the huge mass of cellular genes in the chromosome. In between these two extremes of acute cytocidal and latent infections are various gradations, with viruses that cause somewhat less acute cytocidal infections through to viruses that cause more chronic and persistent infections. A specific disease process called slow-virus diseases occurs toward the chronic end of the disease spectrum. These diseases, of which AIDS is today the most important example, are characterized by a prolonged course after a long silent period and an inexorable progression to death. Some of the mechanisms which operate in slow virus diseases will be discussed in the next chapter.

It is thus important to distinguish between the effects of viruses on host cells from the effects of viral infections and disease at the level of the whole animal or the whole human body. Disease manifestations, as mentioned previously, are a consequence of the type and extent of cellular damage, the sensitivity and functions of the cells and organs involved, as well as the subjective feelings of ill-health. Thus, during the silent phase of infection there may well be acute cytocidal destruction of cells, but it may not be sufficient to cause disease. Similarly, low-grade infection with only subtle structural damage to cells may cause extensive disease because of the body's response or the critical nature of the cells involved. In all viral infections there is a silent phase from the time of infection until the disease mani-festations are felt; this is called the incubation period. During this period of time there is a progressive build-up of viral mass in the body until the stage is reached where there is clinical expression of infection. In infec-tions where the virus is localized to the portals of entry into the body, that is the respiratory tract or the gastro-intestinal tract, this period is short, usually a few days or less. Where a virus is disseminated throughout the body – for example, in the acute infectious diseases of childhood, such as measles, chickenpox and mumps – the incubation period is of the order of a few weeks. With viruses which produce chronic infection, such as hepatitis, the incubation period may be up to a few months. In the slow virus infections this period is often a number of years.

The specificity of viral infections

One of the characteristic features of viruses is their specificity for the cells that they infect – specificity with regard to the species of animal as well as for the organ in the animal (tropism). (Like many things in biology, there are exceptions, for example, the dreaded rabies virus can non-specifically infect all mammalian species.) The specificity of viral infection is, to a large extent but not entirely, due to the specific attachment of the virus to its receptor site on the host cell. Thus, experimentally sticking a human poliomyelitis receptor site onto a mouse cell could render the latter sus-ceptible to poliovirus (although it would not be able to subsequently infect other mouse cells which do not possess the human receptor). There are also additional factors inside a cell that would be inimical to a virus from another species. The same limitations of tropism would apply to infecting cells from different organs in the body. Some viruses may have a relatively wide tropism if their particular receptor site is found in a number of different cell types, and also if the intracellular conditions are widely favourable to that virus. Some viruses are very narrowly tropic; for example, hepatitis A virus will virtually exclusively only infect liver cells, or rotavirus, an important cause of diarrhoeal disease especially in infants, will only infect a certain type of cell in the small intestine.

The interaction between the outermost proteins of the capsid, or envelope, of a virus and the proteins of the cell's receptor site has been likened to that between a lock and key. Subtle changes in these proteins which affect the folding of the protein molecule or the substitution of different amino acid building blocks at critical sites in the protein can affect the interaction between the virus and its receptor site. Also, the presence of soluble proteins of the cell's receptor site in the fluid outside the cell can act as a decoy by attaching to the virus and preventing it, in turn, attaching to the cell's receptor site. This is an important defence mechanism in respiratory secretions for example. The major protective function of the immune system is to produce antibodies directed against the virus which attach to the outermost proteins and thereby prevent them from attaching to the receptor sites. Here too the recognition between the antibody molecule and the protein antigen of the virus is highly specific, and subtle changes in the antigenic composition or structure can affect the attachment and render the immune protection of the host ineffective.

The AIDS virus – HIV

Within this mysterious twilight world of the virus, which straddles the living and the inanimate, is perhaps the most extraordinary of all viruses – the HIV virus. Up until the middle 1970s, no member of the retrovirus family, which had previously been extensively studied in the animal kingdom, was known to occur in humans. This vast knowledge of animal retroviruses, however, had not prepared virologists for what was to emerge with HIV and its related animal immunodeficiency viruses in the 1980s. While it was initially perceived to be a virus of comparative simplicity, relatively small in size, with few genes, as in the case of the other retroviruses, deeper research was soon to demonstrate a virus with an exceedingly complex system to regulate the expression of the few genes responsible for the structure of the virus itself. Research would also soon reveal a virus that was able rapidly to change itself so that even from a single infected individual multiple different variants, now called quasispecies, could be isolated. Also further studies would demonstrate a virus that has a virtually unparalleled ability to evade the immune system of the host.

HIV – where it belongs in the family of viruses

The family of retroviruses (scientifically called Retroviridae) is defined by the presence of the unique enzyme – reverse transcriptase – which facilitates the production of a DNA copy from an RNA genome. All members of the family possess this enzyme and all make DNA copies of their RNA genomes inside the cells that they parasitize. Outside the cell the virus consists of two strands of RNA, but inside the cell the virus genome exists largely in the form of its DNA copy. An essential step in the multiplication of these viruses is the integration of the DNA copy into the chromosome of the host cell. This DNA copy is referred to as a provirus. All members of the retrovirus family have the ability to produce latent infections.

The family Retroviridae consists of a number of viruses, some associated with malignancy in animals and humans; it also includes the virus group called the lentiviruses (lenti = Greek for 'slow'). Within the lentiviruses are found various slow viruses such as the classic visna-maedi virus of sheep and the various animal and human immunodeficiency viruses. All of these viruses share the characteristics of producing slow-virus diseases with many of them affecting cells of the immune system and the brain. More recent research has demonstrated that the biological behaviour of HIV in the human body is far from 'slow', as will be discussed in Chapter 3. For historical reasons it is still classified with the other lentiviruses.

The structure of HIV

Under the electron microscope, HIV appears as a relatively featureless virus, unlike the very characteristic sometimes even striking appearance of many other viruses of humans (Fig. 2.5). It is of medium size, about 100–150 nm in diameter. It is roughly circular in shape, although the pliability of the viral envelope may change the spherical shape to oval or even to a somewhat irregular outline (Fig. 2.6).

The envelope, like all viral envelopes, is partly derived from the cell membrane of the host cell as the virus buds through in the final stages of its replication (Figs. 2.7 and 2.8). The cell membrane component of the envelope is largely composed of lipid or fatty material. On the inside of the envelope there is a protein called the matrix protein which may be visualized as concentrated stained areas called lateral bodies. More importantly, protruding to the outside of the envelope are two viral proteins that are anchored into the outer surface of the envelope. These two envelope proteins are a knob-like protein called gp120 and a smaller spike-like protein called gp41. The 'gp' stands for glycoprotein which is a molecule

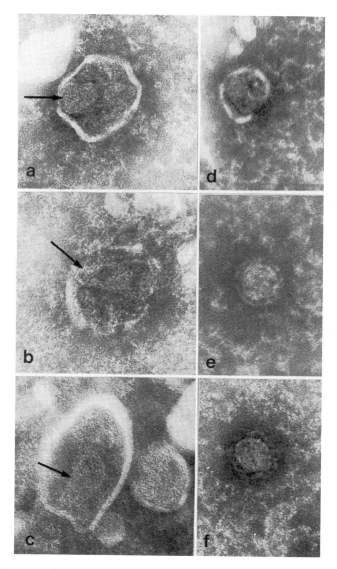

Fig. 2.5 HIV particles under the electron microscope. The conical protein core of a virus is visible in some particles (arrowed). Magnification = 145 000×. (Photograph courtesy of Professor G Lecatsas.)

composed of a carbohydrate component ('glyco-' from 'glukeros' = Greek for 'sweet') and a protein component. The molecular weights of these proteins are 120 000 and 41 000 daltons respectively. (The dalton is the unit of measurement for the mass of a molecule – 1 dalton being approximately

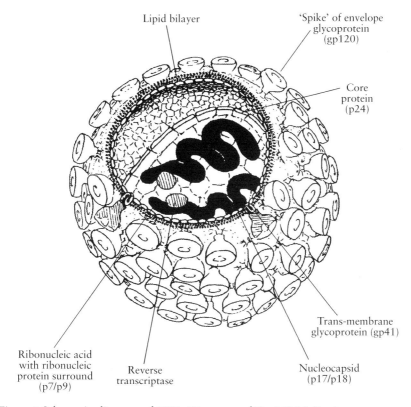

Fig. 2.6 Schematic diagram of HIV. (Courtesy of Dr J G M Sim.)

the mass of a hydrogen atom.) The proteins are critical for the initial attachment of the virus to its cellular receptor site. They are the most important
antigens of the virus, as the antibodies they elicit will be those that could
confer protection by preventing the virus from attaching to the cellular
receptor sites. They will be dealt with in greater detail in Chapter 3.

The inner core of the virus, that is the capsid, which surrounds the
nucleic acid, is characteristically cone-shaped and is the chief feature used
to recognize the virus under the electron microscope. Coiled up within the
core are situated the two strands of RNA together with the enzyme reverse
transcriptase. The main protein of the core of the virus is referred to as p24
(molecular weight 24 000 dalton) and it plays an important diagnostic role,
as will be seen later.

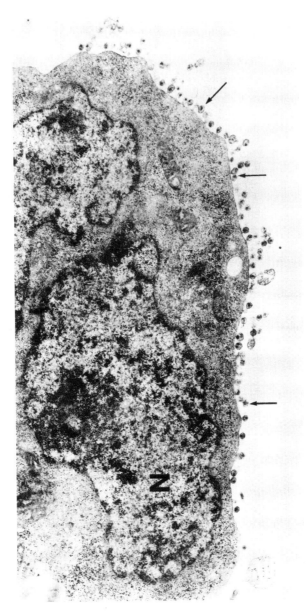

Fig. 2.7 Electron micrograph of HIV-infected lymphocyte showing numerous HIV virus particles that have budded through the cell membrane (arrowed). N = nucleus of the lymphocyte cell. Magnification = 7000×. (Photograph courtesy of Professor G Lecatsas.)

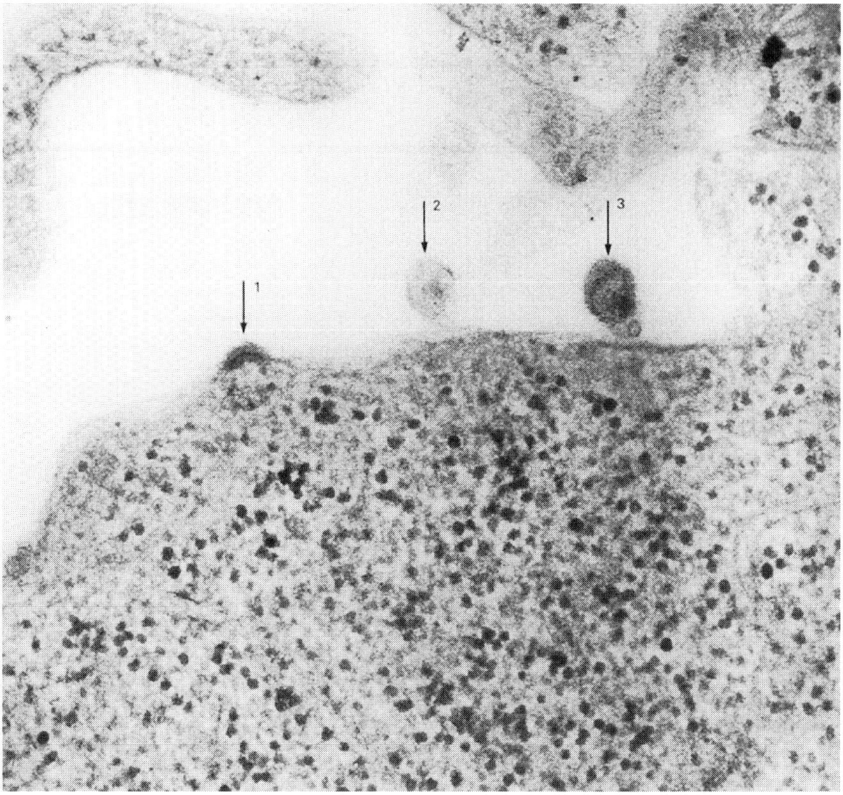

Fig. 2.8 Electron micrograph showing three stages of an HIV virus budding through the cell membrane of an infected lymphocyte. Magnification = 55 000×. (Photograph courtesy of Professor G Lecatsas.)

The genome of HIV

In common with the general pattern of the retroviruses, the genome of HIV is composed of three genes which code for (that is, direct the synthesis of) the inner core proteins, the envelope proteins and the virus enzymes (Fig. 2.9). These genes are named respectively, the *gag* gene (*gag* stands for group *antigen*, as the antigenicity of this protein is the same throughout this group of viruses), the *env* gene (*env* is short for *env*elope) and, thirdly, the *pol* gene (*pol* is short for *pol*ymerase, referring to reverse transcriptase which functions as a polymerase, polymerization being the process of stringing together individual building blocks such as the components of the nucleic acid chain). The *pol* gene also specifies other enzymes: ribonuclease (which cleaves RNA), integrase (which promotes the integration

LIVERPOOL
JOHN MOORES UNIVERSITY
AVRIL ROBARTS LRC
TEL. 0151 231 4022

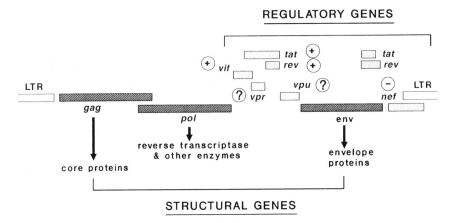

Fig. 2.9 Schematic diagram of the genes of HIV-1

of the nucleic acid into the host cell's chromosome) and protease (which splits proteins into smaller fragments). The proteins which initially come off the manufacturing process and which are specified by each of the three genes are actually composed of larger precursor protein chains that are subsequently cleaved by protease into smaller functional units. For example, the envelope glycoproteins specified by the *env* gene is in fact a much larger molecule called gp160, and it is then split by protease into two smaller functional components of gp120 and gp41. Similarly the products of *gag* gene are also split into three proteins – the matrix protein, the core protein (p24) and another structural protein. Likewise the products of the *pol* gene are split into reverse transcriptase, ribonuclease, integrase and protease.

Also in common with the other retroviruses, HIV possesses at either end of its genome, a segment of nucleic acid called the LTR (long terminal repeat) so-called because the sequence is repeated on either end. This LTR does not itself code for any proteins but regulates and controls whether the three structural genes are turned on to express their proteins, or are turned off. In other words they act as a regulator button for the genome. The LTR of HIV is, however, relatively inefficient as a regulator and its function is largely controlled and augmented by a number of other genes called regulatory genes, of which at least seven have now been described. The complexity of the regulatory apparatus of the HIV genome appears to be vastly out of proportion to the size of the genome which is small even by viral standards, being less than 10 kb in length.

The regulation of HIV

A detailed discussion of the functions of the regulatory system of HIV would be well beyond the scope of this volume. However, a brief description of its components is necessary, as many of these regulatory proteins are now being intensively investigated as possible targets for the design of drugs against HIV.

The regulatory genes can be divided into three groups – positive regulatory genes, negative regulatory genes and regulatory genes whose precise functions still need to be determined (Fig. 2.9). There are four positive regulatory genes, that is genes that produce regulatory proteins which promote the expression of other genes and which positively regulate the formation of viral particles by promoting the production of proteins and the assembly of the components of the virus.

The first of these genes is the *tat* gene (*t*ransactivator of *t*ranscription) which occurs as two separate segments of nucleic acid and produces a protein which attaches itself to a specific site in the LTR (called the TAR site – *ta*t *r*esponsive site) and thereby stimulates the expression of the three structural genes by promoting the transcription of messenger RNA for the manufacture of their proteins. This process of producing a protein to remotely regulate the expression of genes is called transactivation.

Another transactivating protein is produced by the second regulatory gene, called the *rev* gene (*r*egulator of *e*xpression of *v*iral proteins) which functions as a promoter of the export of viral RNA from the nucleus of the cell. This viral RNA acts as a template for the manufacture of the viral structural proteins. The third gene, *vif* (*v*irus *i*nfectivity *f*actor) influences the infectivity of virus particles and also the release of infectious virus from cells. The function of the protein produced by the fourth gene, *vpu* (*v*iral *p*rotein *u*) has not been precisely established but is also known to enhance the production of virus particles by promoting release of infectious virus from cells.

The negative regulator gene, *nef* (*ne*gative *f*actor), produces proteins which act on a section of the LTR called NRE (*n*egative *r*egulatory *e*lement) which in turn sends a message down-regulating viral replication by inhibiting the production of structural proteins. It is needed by the virus for efficient replication. This gene and its product have been the subject of intense research into their possible usage in therapy and also as a diagnostic marker of lower virus activity or latency.

A further two regulatory genes, *vpr* (*v*iral *p*rotein *r*) and *vpt* (*v*iral protein *t*), have also been described, although their function still needs to be elucidated. In HIV-2, a regulatory gene called *vpx* (*v*iral *p*rotein *x*) is present but, again, its function is as yet unknown.

The net effect of this highly complex regulatory machinery is that the expression of the virus is very carefully controlled and it facilitates the switch from being in a latent state, where the expression of its genes is switched off, to a highly active and rapidly multiplying state, where there may be exuberant production of viral particles.

A most important consequence of the regulatory apparatus relates to the fact that the effects of these regulatory proteins are not confined to the genes of HIV, but they may also modify the expression of cellular genes. Thus, the activation of cellular genes by transactivating proteins from HIV may well have an important bearing on the development of the tumours which are of such importance in AIDS. Similarly, transactivating proteins made by cells or by other viruses may also regulate and activate the expression of HIV genes. This is thought to be the mechanism by which, for example, the activation of cells of the immune system (which house HIV) may, as a result of immune stimulation, in turn activate the virus. Also, concurrent infection with viruses, especially herpes viruses or HTLV-I, are known to be potent activators of HIV.

The envelope glycoproteins

The two envelope glycoproteins, because of their critical role at the important initial steps of infection (that is, attachment and penetration into the cell) and for the production of antibodies which neutralize the virus, have been particularly intensively studied. The gp120 protein consists of a chain of amino acid building blocks folded to form the characteristic knob-shaped structure. Within the chain there are five segments where the amino acid sequence remains fairly constant in different isolates of the virus, and these constant segments are denoted as C_1 to C_5. In addition, there are five segments where the sequence of amino acids varies quite markedly from isolate to isolate, and these variable segments are denoted as V_1 to V_5. The third variable segment, V_3, also called the V_3 loop, is the subject of great interest as it is this segment which has been shown to elicit neutralizing antibodies and which is also specifically responsible for the initial attachment to the receptor site of susceptible cells (called the CD4 receptor site). The gp120 knob is covered by a sugar coating which protects it from the immune response of the host, although the V_3 loop of gp120 protrudes beyond this coating in order to make contact with the cells to be infected (Fig. 2.10). A second portion of the gp120 which is left uncovered by the sugar coating is a series of hollow depressions formed

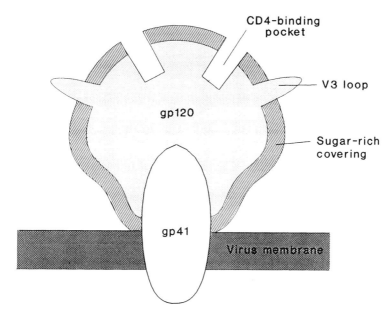

Fig 2.10 Schematic diagram of the structure of the envelope glycoprotein of HIV.

by the folding of portions of the protein chain to bind to the CD4 protein, the so-called CD4 binding pockets.

The gp41 spikes are also referred to as transmembrane proteins, as they are inserted through the lipid envelope and do not protrude far beyond the outside of the envelope. The function of this glycoprotein is to fuse the envelope of the virus to the membrane of the host cell, thus facilitating the entry of the virus into the cell for the further steps of replication.

Replication of HIV

The steps in the replication process of HIV have been intensively studied, as each stage in the cycle of replication may provide an opportunity for the design of an effective antiviral drug (see Figs. 6.2 and 6.3).

The first event to occur in replication is the attachment of the virus to the host cell via the V3 loop of gp120. This attachment process causes structural changes to occur in gp120 that expose cleavage sites which can then be attacked by enzymes, causing it to split open. The effect of this is to expose the gp41 which is otherwise covered over and masked by gp120. The gp41 can now cause fusion to take place between the viral envelope and the cell membrane, following which the core of the virus enters into the cell. Once inside the cell the core capsid protein breaks open releasing the two strands of the virus RNA. The reverse transcriptase then makes a DNA copy from each of these strands and these copies are then integrated into the host cell chromosome. Messenger RNA to control the production of the proteins of the virus as well as RNA, which will be used for the progeny virus, are copied from the integrated viral genes. The final steps involve the assembly of the protein and the nucleic acid components into progeny virus particles which are released from the cell and these are then able to infect new cells and repeat the process.

The replication cycle is, of course, very carefully regulated and controlled not only by the viral regulatory genes but also by influences of the cell and possibly also other viruses, as described above. The whole cycle may thus proceed fairly rapidly, or it may be prolonged, or it may even be arrested, usually immediately after integration when the virus may remain in a latent state for extended periods of time.

Variability of HIV

One of the most important properties of HIV from a clinical point of view is its variability. The variability is due mainly to the inaccuracy of its genetic copying mechanism and the proneness of this mechanism to make errors. During each replication cycle of the virus about 10–20 mistakes are made. In general terms RNA viruses tend to be more variable than DNA viruses because the RNA replication mechanism does not have a facility to effect repairs to the growing nucleic acid chain, as is the case with the DNA replication mechanism. In addition to this the enzyme reverse transcriptase is itself particularly error-prone and is not meticulously faithful in making a DNA copy from the RNA template. Errors may creep in at any of the three stages of RNA replication, with each stage multiplying the mistake even further.

Mutations which affect the sequence of the nucleic acid may or may not, initially, affect the virus in any way. The effect of the substitution of a single nucleotide in a sequence would depend on how critical the site is in the particular gene affected. Ultimately, however, accumulation of these point mutations will eventually give rise to sufficiently important changes in the proteins produced from these genes to cause functional changes in the virus. With the rapidity of change that occurs in HIV, it is small wonder that different strains of virus arise in individuals with established HIV infections. These strains have significant differences in important biological properties; for example, their rate of growth, their virulence in terms of ability to kill cells, their sensitivity to antibodies produced by the host, the antigenicity of their proteins and their ability to evade the host's immune response. Because of the substantive differences in these isolates, they are referred to as quasispecies. The variability of HIV plays a major role in the natural history of HIV infection and HIV disease, as will be discussed more fully in the next chapter.

In addition to these variations of the virus found in a particular infected individual, there are a number of different subtypes of HIV which predominate in different parts of the world. To date some 10 subtypes, also referred to as clades, have been described and designated as A–J. Subtype B is the predominant subtype in Europe and North America and subtype C in southern Africa and India.

The isolation and growth of HIV

Techniques used for the isolation and propagation of HIV have, in principle, differed little from those pioneered by Montagnier and Gallo in the early- to mid-1980s. The cell cultures used are usually derived from human lymphocytes and may either be lymphocytes extracted from the blood of healthy donors or certain cell lines prepared from malignant lymphoid tumours or leukaemic material (Fig. 2.11). Cell cultures of malignant origin do have the advantage of convenience because these cells have an indefinite life span and can be stored in ultra-low-temperature freezers and then

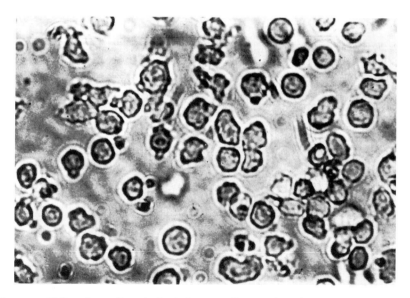

Fig 2.11 Cell culture line derived from malignant lymphocytes, used for the isolation and growth of HIV.

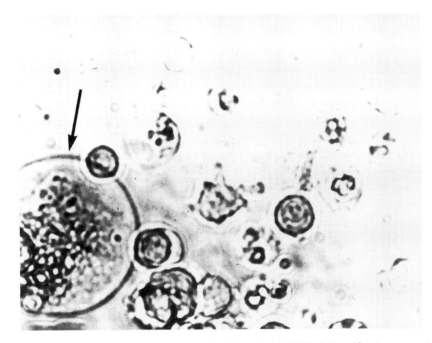

Fig 2.12 Syncytium (giant cell, arrowed) infected with HIV. (Magnification 400×.)

thawed and used as and when needed. As tumour cells are by nature rapidly multiplying, they are already in a state of activation and are receptive to infection with HIV. Lymphocytes derived from blood donors, however, require to be artificially activated and this is done using various lymphocyte-activating materials.

In cell culture HIV often causes relatively easily recognizable pathological changes in the cells that it infects. Degenerating cells characteristically balloon out and may also fuse with each other to form syncytia, which are clearly visible under the microscope (Fig. 2.12). The ability to cause balloon degeneration and syncytia formation is a function of some strains (quasispecies) of HIV and may be absent in others. Indirect techniques are also used to detect the presence of HIV growing in cell cultures, especially when these visible signs of infection do not occur; for example, by the demonstration of p24 antigen in the fluid medium in which the cells are suspended, or by the measurement of the enzyme reverse transcriptase.

The ability to isolate and propagate HIV has improved greatly over the years. Initially the isolation rate for known positive human material was in the order of only 10–20%. This has now increased to 80% or even higher.

The stability of HIV

The envelopes of viruses are generally delicate structures that are quite easily damaged and disrupted when the virus is exposed to the outside environment. They are also fairly sensitive to heat and, being composed of lipid (fatty) material, are vulnerable to the action of detergents such as found in soaps, as well as lipid solvents such as alcohol and ether. Although there are some exceptionally stable enveloped viruses, such as hepatitis B, as a general rule enveloped viruses tend to be considerably more delicate and unable to survive outside the body for nearly as long as the more robust non-enveloped viruses. The enveloped HIV virus is no exception and it is as fragile as the average enveloped virus.

Questions surrounding the stability of HIV have been very fertile ground for alarmists and sensationalists and a great deal of incorrect information has been propagated about the alleged stability of the virus.

There are two ways of ascertaining the stability of the virus and its ability to survive in various conditions. Probably the more meaningful way is the epidemiological one; in other words, drawing conclusions from available information on which kinds of individuals have been infected by various routes of transmission. This information points very strongly against the virus being spread other than by the accepted routes of sexual transmission and by blood exchange, and there is certainly no evidence that the virus is disseminated to any observable extent by contact with inanimate surfaces, through the air or via ingestion. Also, one can experimentally measure the survival of known amounts of virus in various environmental conditions. However, it must be borne in mind that these experimental evaluations are carried out on virus grown in culture under laboratory conditions. These conditions may well favour the virus to a greater extent than natural conditions would. Also, artificially high doses of virus are used in experimental studies, usually considerably higher than would be encountered in the vast majority of natural situations.

Under these experimental conditions, HIV has been shown to survive in dechlorinated tap water for up to 11 days – of the same order as other enveloped viruses such as herpes simplex but considerably shorter than the robust non-enveloped viruses such as polio. In chlorinated tap water and certainly in the highly chlorinated water used in swimming pools and Jacuzzis, the virus would probably rapidly be inactivated within hours.

In the air the virus is rapidly inactivated apart from the very high doses generated in laboratories growing high concentrations of virus. In the latter situation aerosols of virus suspended in organic material may well survive for hours and do constitute a hazard to laboratory workers.

The survival of virus on inanimate surfaces is similar to that of other enveloped viruses. If the virus is in some organic material and is dried at room temperature on surfaces, it may be detectable for up to seven days.

Similar survival times have been observed for virus in blood specimens kept at room temperature and also for virus in the bodies of individuals who have died of AIDS.

HIV, as with the other enveloped viruses, is sensitive to heat, and temperatures of 56°C for 30 minutes have been considered adequate for the inactivation of virus in biological products derived from blood; for example, clotting factor used for treating haemophiliacs. Boiling temperature would undoubtedly inactivate the virus within minutes and can be used, when necessary, to sterilize instruments, provided organic material has been removed.

It is, however, critically important to reiterate that these survival times are based on experimental observations using high doses of tissue-culture-grown virus suspended in tissue culture fluid with added serum for protection of the virus. Such conditions would very rarely be mimicked in nature. No studies have been reported where infectious virus has been isolated from surfaces in the vicinity of AIDS patients, or toilet seats and door handles touched by infected individuals. Similarly, extensive studies of family members of infected persons living under the same roof have not revealed any evidence of virus transmission, other than sexually, suggesting that the virus cannot survive on inanimate surfaces to a sufficient degree to be able to effectively transmit infection. This will be dealt with more fully in Chapter 4.

HIV is also fairly rapidly and easily inactivated by chemicals used for disinfection. The envelope is susceptible to detergents and soap is effective in inactivating HIV. Alcohols, especially a 70% aqueous suspension of alcohol, will inactivate HIV if it is in water but if it is water-free alcohol it may not be effective as it may not be able to penetrate sufficiently into the virus. Alcohol also requires at least a minute or two to penetrate adequately for it to reliably inactivate HIV. Thus, for cleaning surfaces and mopping up spills, chlorine, contained in household bleach (diluted 1 in 10 to 1 in 100), is effective, provided most organic material is removed. Other disinfectants such as glutaraldehyde- and formaldehyde-containing compounds are highly effective and are used in medical and laboratory settings. Hydrogen peroxide is effective for small objects such as contact lenses.

The choice of disinfectant would usually depend on what needs to be disinfected and the type of contamination. However, in general terms, heat sterilization is to be preferred to chemical.

Conclusion

The HIV virus is truly a remarkable infective agent and is in many ways a unique pathogen in humans. Many of its properties are such that antiviral therapy or vaccine development are peculiarly difficult to design, as shall be seen in subsequent chapters. Nevertheless, there is nothing mysterious or supernatural about the survival or transmissibility of the virus. It is, in fact, very poorly transmissible by viral standards and relatively labile, in keeping with its being an enveloped virus.

3

The disease mechanisms of HIV

We have seen in the previous chapter how truly extraordinary an agent the HIV virus is. On the one hand it is of the utmost simplicity, having only three genes available to specify its structure, but, on the other hand, it possesses an exceedingly complex regulatory mechanism to control the expression of these genes. It is also, as we have seen, a virus which is of low transmissibility and not inconsiderable delicacy. At the same time it is also capable of causing one of the most devastating diseases of humankind which, after a decade and a half of some of the most intense research efforts, has seen relatively little measurable success towards a distant goal of a cure. How does a virus, which at first glance does not appear to be a highly formidable foe, persist in the body for such long periods of time and continue multiplying and progressively causing more and more damage until a fatal outcome is reached? Why is it that the immensely powerful immune system of the body, an organ system which has evolved over millennia of challenges from a wide variety of infectious and non-infectious invaders to become an exceedingly effective defender of the body against micro-organisms apparently far more virulent than the AIDS virus, now appear to be powerless against such a seemingly puny foe?

As the immune system and its functions are so critical to the understanding of the pathogenesis (the steps taken along the path to pathology, or disease), it may be as well to first consider some of the basic elements of this complex system.

The immune system

Higher animals and humans have evolved, through millions of years of contact with invading organisms, an extremely effective and involved system of tissues and organs for defence against potentially pathogenic intruders. The power and the efficacy of this system can be gauged by the fact that there is a parallel evolutionary process on the part of micro-organisms, which mutate rapidly and have a far greater ability for adaptive change to escape from the effects of the immune system. Nevertheless, even though animals and Man are continually in contact with a sea of micro-organisms, many of them potentially pathogenic, disease is a rare event and when it does occur an intact and functioning immune system is able to effectively eliminate the organism and effect a cure in the vast majority of cases.

The structure of the immune system

Essentially the immune system consists of three functional sections: there is an afferent arm, that part of the immune system which receives the intruding organism or foreign material and processes the relevant message for conveyance to the second section, the management section. The latter then administers the appropriate and effective set of responses which are conveyed to the third section, the efferent arm of the immune system that is that part which will deal with and get rid of the intruder. An offshoot of the management system is a memory data bank for storage of details of the intruder. Should it be encountered again the response is very much accelerated and the intruder is dispatched very much more rapidly, usually even before any clinical signs or symptoms of a potential disease are manifest.

The cells involved in the immune system are presented in Fig. 3.1 and Table 3.1.

The afferent arm

The afferent arm of the immune system consists essentially of cells called macrophages (makros = Greek for 'large' and phag = Greek for 'eat'), also called phagocytes (-cyte = cell). Macrophages are found throughout the body; in tissues they are called tissue macrophages, but are often also given specific names in various organs. In the bloodstream are found the circulating macrophages, usually called monocytes (a member of the family of white blood cells). In the brain, macrophages are referred to as microglial cells ('-glial' refers to brain tissue). Macrophages, whether tissue macrophages or monocytes or microglial cells, are derived from the same

LIVERPOOL JOHN MOORES UNIVERSITY
LEARNING SERVICES

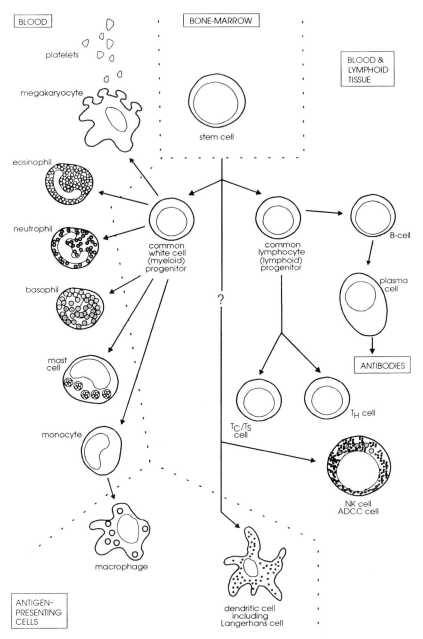

Fig. 3.1 Schematic diagram of the cells involved in the immune system. T_C (or CTL) = cytotoxic T-lymphocyte; T_S = T-suppressor lymphocyte; T_H = T-helper lymphocyte; NK = natural killer cell; ADCC = antibody-dependent cytotoxic cells. (See also Table 3.1.)

Table 3.1 *Cells of the immune system*

Cell type	Function
Macrophage	1. Ingests and removes foreign material. 2. Antigen-presenting cell. Presents foreign antigens (proteins) to the immune system. 3. Produces a variety of regulatory chemicals that function as intercullular messengers (cytokines).
Monocytes	1. Give rise to macrophages. 2. Have macrophage-like functions in the blood – the pair are often referred to together as monocyte/macrophage.
Dendritic cells	1. Antigen-presenting cell. 2. Nurturing function for lymphocytes.
T-helper lymphocyte (T_H)	1. Central regulatory cell of the immune system. Interconnects with other cells by means of cytokine messengers.
T-suppressor lymphocyte (T_S)	1. Negative regulator cell – negative feedback function to prevent excessive activity of cells of the immune system.
Cytotoxic T-lymphocyte (T_c) *or* (CTL)	1. Effector cell of cellular immunity – attacks and destroys infected or malignant cells. 2. Specifically activated by a foreign antigen. 3. Activity is specific to cells of the same species because it recognizes both the specific antigen and also MHC II antigen on target cell.
Natural killer cell (NK)	1. Effector cell of cellular immunity 2. Attacks and destroys cells with foreign antigens on them from infection (viral) or malignancy. 3. Not specifically activated – always present.
Kller cell (K)	1. Effector cell of cellular immunity 2. Recognizes the Fc portion of antibody molecule attached to antigens on surface of infected cell. 3. Not specifically activated – always present.
B-lymphocyte	1. Major cell of humoral immunity. 2. Changes into plasma cell to produce antibody. 3. Retains a 'memory' of antigens it has experienced for more rapid response on re-exposure to same antigen.
Plasma cell	1. Produces antibody.
Neutrophil	1. Attacks invading bacteria by ingesting them and producing chemicals that are antimicrobial.
Eosinophil	1. Primary defence against parasite invasion. 2. Activated by allergic responses.
Basophil and mast cell	1. Removal of foreign proteins that can cause allergic responses. 2. Tissue repair.

Platelets produced from their precursor cell, the megakaryocyte, although derived from the same white cell progenitor, are concerned with blood clotting and are not part of the immune system.

lineage. The function of the macrophages, as the name suggests, is to 'eat' or ingest foreign material, including micro-organisms and clear them from the body. The foreign material, once ingested, is acted on by various enzymes inside the macrophage and it is then 'presented' in an appropriately processed form to the management team of the immune system. The cells that are mainly involved in presenting foreign antigen to the immune system are the dendritic cells, also known as the professional antigen-presenting cells. They are found throughout the body but especially in the bloodstream, in the lymph nodes and in mucous membranes. In the latter site these cells are called Langerhans cells and they are of direct importance in HIV infection, as they are important vehicles for transporting HIV from the peripheral mucous membranes of the genital tract centrally to the lymph nodes (see Chapter 4).

The central management

The immune system is managed by lymphocytes which are found in the family of white cells in the bloodstream (where they usually constitute some 20–40% of the total number of white cells), as well as in the lymphoid organ system. This system is located in lymph glands, in organs such as the liver and spleen, and in various aggregates of lymphoid tissue; for example, in the tonsils, in the wall of the gut, inside the abdominal cavity and elsewhere. When first described by the early histologists, lymphocytes were seen to be small, rather featureless blood cells and were assumed to be homogeneous in structure and function (Fig. 3.2). However, because they were also found in lymph nodes and lymphoid tissue, they were suspected to play some role in immune function. Later on morphological subdivisions of lymphocytes were recognized, but it was the advent of techniques for the demonstration of different surface antigens on lymphocytes, which could act as labels or markers, which provided the basis for a rational and functional classification of lymphocytes. This, together with advanced immunochemical technologies that permitted the identification of the numerous biochemical messenger molecules called cytokines, through which the different component cells of the immune system are able to communicate with each other, opened up the understanding of how the immune system regulates and controls itself and puts into action its immune response.

Lymphocytes are subdivided into two main functional groups (demonstrable by the specific markers on the cell surface), T-lymphocytes (so-called because the precursors of these cells are processed and educated for their functional role by the thymus gland situated in the upper chest) and B-lymphocytes (because their precursors are processed in birds through an

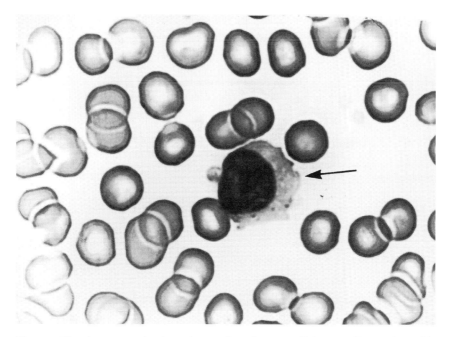

Fig. 3.2 Blood smear stained to show a lymphocyte cell (arrowed) together with numerous non-nucleated smaller red blood cells. (Magnification 1500×.)

organ called the Bursa of Fabricius and in mammals, it is thought, through the bone marrow) (Fig. 3.3A). The T-lymphocytes are themselves subdivided, also on functional grounds and on demonstrable specific cell surface markers that allow them to be visually identified, into various subtypes, two of the most prominent being CD4 and CD8 lymphocytes (Fig. 3.3B). The CD4 lymphocyte is labelled by its surface marker, the CD4 antigen, and these lymphocytes are often also called T4 lymphocytes. They are the main regulatory cells of the immune system and interact with both the afferent and the efferent arms of the immune system. Because of this role they are also often called T-helper lymphocytes or T_H lymphocytes (thus T-4 lymphocytes, T_H lymphocytes and CD4 lymphocytes are all synonymous).

The CD8 lymphocyte has a corresponding CD8 antigen on its surface and is also called a T-8 lymphocyte. This lymphocyte has the opposing effect to the T-helper lymphocyte and thus acts to balance it. The CD8 lymphocyte is therefore also called a T-suppressor lymphocyte or T_S lymphoctye (thus T-8 lymphocyte, T_S lymphocyte and CD8 lymphocyte are all synonymous). Under normal circumstances there are approximately twice as many CD4 lymphocytes as there are CD8 lymphocytes.

(A)

B
cells

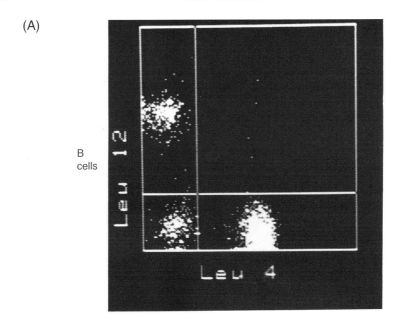

(B)

CD8
lymphocytes

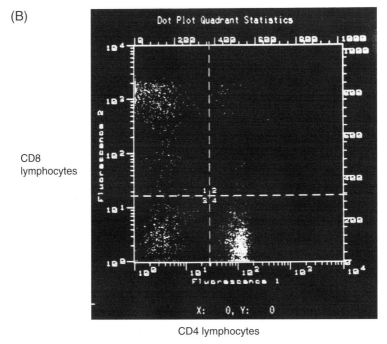

CD4 lymphocytes

Fig. 3.3 Picture of the screen of a flow cytometer (see Fig. 5.10) used for the quantitation of T- and B-cells (A) and CD4 and CD8 lymphocytes (B).

The efferent arm

The efferent arm of the immune response consists of a number of cellular components. Firstly, there are T-lymphocytes that, like T-suppressor lymphocytes, also have CD8 markers on their surface, which are called cytotoxic T-lymphocytes (CTL). When activated as part of the immune response they will, as their name implies, kill cells infected by a particular micro-organism such as a virus, as one way of eliminating the intruding organism. CTLs also attack viruses by producing soluble proteins which inhibit the replication of viruses inside infected cells. CTLs, therefore, play a crucial role in the body's immune response to viral infection.

There are, in addition, two types of lymphocytes which are related to each other but are not T-lymphocytes. Natural killer (NK) cells circulate in the bloodstream and recognize and eliminate cells infected by viruses as well as malignant cells as they arise. Killer (K) cells also circulate in the bloodstream and attach to antibody molecules which are themselves specifically attached to antigens on the surface of infected cells; they are therefore also called antibody-dependent cytotoxic cells (ADCC). Both the NK and K cells differ functionally from the CTLs in that they are not elicited in response to a specific antigen, but they can be activated by various products in the body; for example, interferon and other lymphokines (materials produced by activated lymphocytes). These three cells form the cellular effector arm of the immune response.

The other component of the effector arm of the immune response involves activities of soluble proteins called antibodies which are produced by the B-lymphocytes. When the B-lymphocyte receives the signal from the T-helper lymphocyte, it undergoes certain structural and other changes to become a plasma cell, whose function is to produce antibodies specifically directed against the antigens of the intruding micro-organism or foreign material. This component of the effector immune response is referred to as the humoral immune response, using the word 'humor' for its meaning of 'fluid' (humorem = Latin for 'moisture') to indicate that antibody proteins are in the fluid component as distinct from the cellular component of blood.

The immune system at work

The workings of the immune system, therefore, commence with the ingestion of foreign protein material by macrophages and dendritic cells. Once inside these antigen-presenting cells the foreign protein is broken down into small pieces by the cells' enzymes and it is then attached onto

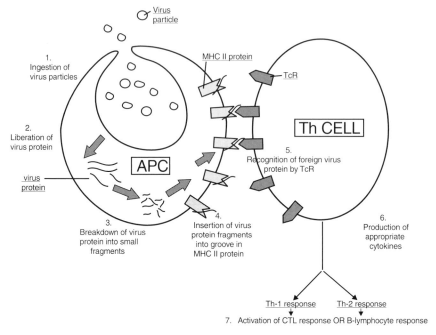

Fig. 3.4 Schematic representation of presentation of virus antigens to the immune system; APC = antigen-presenting cell (dendritic cell or macrophage), Th = T-helper cell (CD4 lymphocyte), TcR = T-cell receptor, MHC = major histocompatibility complex protein.

a cellular protein called MHC II (major histocompatibility class II). (The MHC proteins are used as identifying labels by the immune system which can then recognize that a particular cell belongs to the individual and is not foreign. The MHC class I protein is involved in CTL recognition, as will be discussed later in this chapter.) The MHC II protein together with the fragment of foreign protein is then transported to the outer membrane of the cell and protrudes from the surface of the cell. The CD4 lympho-cyte has a corresponding surface protein protruding from its cell membrane called the T-cell receptor (TcR) which is able to recognize and attach to the foreign protein inserted into a groove of the MHC II molecule of the antigen-presenting cell (Fig. 3.4). The recognition and attachment step triggers a series of biochemical reactions in the CD4 cell causing it to produce small biologically potent proteins called cytokines which act as messengers to the effector cells of the immune system. These cytokines, of which an ever increasing number are being described, constitute an extra-ordinarily complex system of signals to various cells of the immune system.

With regard to the effector immune response, two main groups of cytokines are produced. The one group activates the cellular immune response, i.e. CTLs, and the other the humoral immune response, i.e. the B-lymphocytes. The cytokine response for CTL activation is also called a Th1 response and that for the B-lymphocyte activation a Th2 response (Th for T-helper cell). Thus, both the cellular and the humoral arms of the immune response are activated.

The cellular effector arm

The major component of the cellular immune response is the CTL. Activated CTLs need to recognize those cells which have been infected by, for example, viruses. In the case of CTL recognition it is the MHC I protein which is involved in the identification of the cell. During replication of viruses inside the cell, fragments of viral protein are inserted into a groove in the MHC I molecule and transported to the surface of the infected cell. CTL cells are then able to recognize and attach to the MHC I molecule containing the fragment of viral protein and it is this which triggers the CTL to either destroy the infected cell, or alternatively to produce soluble proteins which inhibit further viral replication (Fig. 3.5).

The humoral (antibody) effector arm

Activation of B-lymphocytes by the Th2 cytokines causes them to undergo the structural and functional changes necessary for them to become plasma cells, which produce antibodies in the bloodstream and in the secretions of the various mucous membranes of the body. Antibodies are globulin proteins in serum and in various secretions of the body, and are of five types. The two most important types of globulins in serum are called IgM and IgG (Ig = immunoglobulin). IgM is produced first in response to infection and usually appears some 14 days after infection, although in chronic and slow infections this may be considerably prolonged. This is followed about a week later by IgG which remains present for years after infection, while the IgM decreases and then disappears, usually after about three months. Another type of immunoglobulin, IgA, is found in the secretions of the body's mucous membranes as well as serum.

The immunoglobulins neutralize viruses and other micro-organisms by clumping them or coating them, thus preventing them from attaching to their specific receptor sites, or, in the case of enveloped viruses, they may directly disrupt the envelope and thus inactivate the virus. They may also, by coating viruses, make them more 'palatable' for ingestion by macrophages.

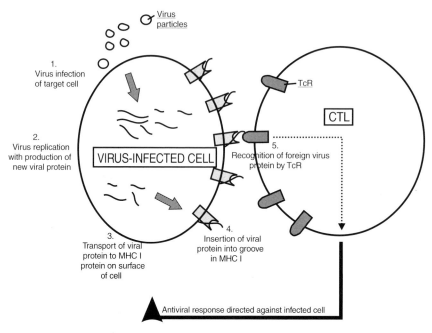

Fig. 3.5 Schematic representation of recognition of viral-infected target cell and antiviral CTL response; CTL = cytotoxic T-lymphocyte, TcR = T-cell receptor, MHC = major histocompatibility complex protein.

The specificity of the immune system

One of the essential features of the immune response is its specificity. The recognition of the protein structure by effector CTL cells or by antibody molecules is crucial to the success of the immune response. This recognition is highly specific to the antigen that elicited the response, i.e. that was originally presented to the CD4 lymphocyte, and even subtle changes in the antigen can abrogate the efficacy of the immune response. Diagnostic techniques that rely on the specificity of this interaction of antigen and antibody are called serological techniques, and are usually used to detect specific antibodies using a known antigen and in this way identify infections with a particular virus. The converse is also used in diagnostic laboratories, that is to detect specific antigens using known antibodies as reagents (see Chapter 5).

It is into this powerful, complex and highly efficient system that the apparently frail HIV virus intrudes. Initially it is met by a vigorous CTL onslaught which eliminates most, but not all, of the virus. The remnant virus eventually establishes itself and then progressively and relentlessly overcomes the immune system and eventually the patient. To understand how this occurs we must relate how certain of the specific properties of the virus that have been discussed enable it to overcome the formidable immune system and cause progressive and ultimately lethal disease.

Properties of HIV related to virus–host interactions

The CD4 protein as a receptor for HIV

One of the major receptor sites in the body for HIV is the CD4 protein which is a surface antigen found on a number of cells. It is present in great profusion and is indeed the identifying surface marker of the T-helper lymphocyte, which is a prime target cell for the virus. This is particularly unfortunate as the T-helper lymphocyte is one of the most crucial cells in the body because of its key functional role as the essential regulator and controller of the immune system. It is therefore not surprising that there is such severe immunosuppression following the profound depletion of the T-helper lymphocytes.

The CD4 antigen is also found on a number of other cells in the body, some of which also have an important bearing on the course of HIV infection. A cell of great importance with respect to the transmission of HIV, and also as a conveyer of the virus in the body, is the Langerhans cell named after the nineteenth century pathologist, Paul Langerhans (who, incidentally, discovered and described these cells when a medical student). The Langerhans cell is a member of the dendritic cell system, the professional antigen-presenting cells of the body. The dendritic cells also have a role supporting and nurturing the T-lymphocytes. Langerhans cells are found in the skin and in the mucous membranes of the body, and in particular profusion in the mucosa of the female and male genitalia. They circulate continually between the peripheral mucous membranes and the CD4 lymphocytes found in lymph nodes and other lymphoid tissue. They are therefore of particular importance in HIV infection, as they probably constitute the major vehicle for transporting HIV from the mucous membranes to the lymphocytes in the lymph nodes. The Langerhans cell may well be the key to understanding how HIV is transmitted across the intact genital mucous membrane. (Earlier concepts of the sexual transmission of HIV put forward that the virus could only be transmitted via blood exchange and that breaks in the mucous membrane of the genitalia were obligatory to allow for blood contact between individuals. This was refuted by later animal experiments as well as by observations of HIV transmission by artificial insemination, which established that sexual transmission could occur across an intact mucous membrane.) Once the Langerhans cell is infected in the mucous membrane, its natural physiological migration route transports it to the T-lymphocytes in lymphoid tissue where it would function as an antigen-presenting cell. In HIV-infected individuals, therefore, the Langerhans cell presents the HIV virus to its natural target cell, the CD4 lymphocyte, which becomes infected and ultimately is killed by the virus.

A third cell type of importance to HIV infection is the monocyte/macrophage cell which also has CD4 antigen on its surface but not in such abundance as the T-helper lymphocyte and is relatively resistant to its killing effect. Monocytes also have another important role in HIV infection in that they convey virus in a Trojan horse fashion into the central nervous system. They constantly circulate to the central nervous system where they change into microglial cells which, as mentioned previously, are the macrophage equivalents in the brain.

A second receptor (co-receptor) for HIV

Although the CD4 molecule has long been established to be a receptor site for HIV, it has also been recognized for a number of years that an additional receptor site on the cell is necessary for the entry of the virus into the cell. In 1996, scientists at the National Institutes of Health in the USA discovered that the alternative receptor site for HIV is another surface protein, which functions physiologically as the receptor site for a subgroup of cytokines called chemokines. By adding these soluble chemokines to cell cultures, they are able to effectively block the attachment of HIV to cells even though the CD4 receptors are still present and available. Two kinds of co-receptors have been identified – one is required by macrophage-tropic (M-tropic) variants of HIV to infect macrophages and is called the CCR-5 receptor, and the other is required by T-lymphotropic (T-tropic) variants of HIV and is called the CXCR-4 receptor.

The importance of the discovery of these co-receptors is that it may lead to opportunities for the development of antiviral agents that can block attachment of the virus to them. (Unfortunately the natural chemokines cannot be used therapeutically as their physiological role is to regulate the inflammatory process and administration to a patient could aggravate the inflammatory response. Derivatives of these chemokines would need to be developed for possible therapeutic use.) The dependence of the M-tropic and the T-tropic variants of HIV on their respective co-receptors could help explain the shift in their predominance in the early and later stages of infection, respectively, as a result of viral mutation. Perhaps the most exciting consequence of the discovery of these co-receptors is that it provides an explanation for the apparent natural resistance of certain individuals to HIV infection. Investigators from a number of countries in the world have identified individuals who persist in high-risk practices and are consequently repetitively exposed to the virus, yet remain free of infection. These individuals have been identified amongst homosexual men in the USA, female prostitutes in Kenya and intravenous drug abusers in Europe. A worldwide population study has revealed that 11% of Caucasians, but a far lower percentage of other races, have a mutation in their genes for the CCR-5 chemokine receptor and are consequently resistant to HIV.

Entry of virus into cells

The postulated route of entry of HIV into cells is illustrated in Fig. 3.6. The initial step is the attachment of the gp120 envelope protein of the virus onto its specific receptor site, the CD4 protein (point 1). This initial step then causes structural changes to the surface of the virus, allowing it to attach to the co-receptor which brings the gp41 protein of HIV into closer contact with the cell membrane (point 2). The gp41 can then mediate fusion of the viral envelope with the cell membrane (point 3), permitting the virus to penetrate into the cell and commence replicating (point 4).

How does HIV kill cells?

Recent studies of the dynamics of viral replication and the compensatory regeneration of the CD4 lymphocytes have revealed a picture of intense struggle with some 5% of the total population of the CD4 cells (about 2000 million cells) being destroyed by billions of viral particles. The precise mechanism or mechanisms of this massive cellular destruction had not been established at the time of writing. Direct and indirect mechanisms have been postulated. HIV could directly kill cells in two possible ways: firstly, by a process called apoptosis which means the programming of cells to undergo a number of biochemical changes leading to their death. Apoptosis is a mechanism used physiologically by the body to rid itself of unwanted cell clones in the immune system. A second possibility is that of the superantigen mechanism. A superantigen is an antigen which is able to bypass the normal antigen presentation mechanism outlined earlier. The superantigen can directly couple the antigen-presenting cell to the CD4 lymphocyte, thus triggering off an abnormally vigorous pathological immune response which destroys cells.

HIV infection could also result in cell death by an indirect pathway whereby the immune response kills the body's own cells. As CTLs recognize HIV-infected cells and destroy them, it is not surprising that the

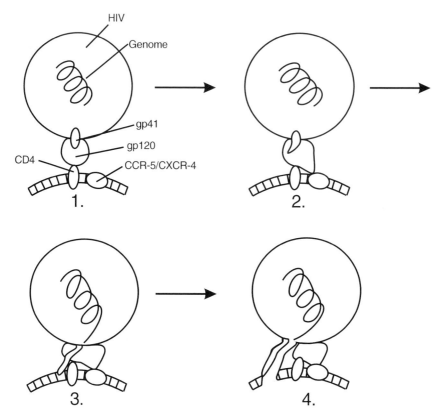

Fig. 3.6 Schematic representation of steps in the infection of a macrophage by HIV.
1. Attachment of gp120 of HIV to CD4 receptor site of cell. 2. Attachment
of gp120 to co-receptor CCR-5 on macrophages or CXCR-4 on lymphocytes.
3. Attachment of gp41 to cell membrane, which mediates fusion of viral envelope
with cell membrane. 4. Penetration of viral genome into cell to commence replication.

infected CD4 lymphocyte would become an obvious target and there is
indeed mounting evidence that the CD4 depletion is to some extent due to
destruction by the CTLs as part of the cellular immune response to the virus.

HIV and the central nervous system

Another apparent enigma of HIV infection is its effect on the central nervous system. In advanced AIDS, and certainly in clinical AIDS dementia,
there is a marked depletion of neural tissue, and at post-mortem severe
shrinkage of the brain is seen, attesting to the extensive destruction of brain
tissue. Yet, HIV has never been convincingly demonstrated to infect neu-

rones and has not been isolated from these cells in patients. Furthermore, neurones have little or no CD4 antigen on their surfaces.

Damage and destruction of neurones is generally thought to be a secondary result of infection of microglial cells and the subsequent release of various cytokines and other active inflammatory molecules, especially substances called kinins which are largely responsible for the pathological consequences of the inflammatory response. These materials may also be responsible for a number of the general effects of HIV disease, such as wasting, chronic pyrexia, chronic diarrhoea and premature ageing.

Consequences of the variability of HIV

As discussed in the previous chapter, HIV is intrinsically a highly variable virus with an error rate of some 10–20 per replication cycle. With hundreds of millions of virus particles being produced daily, it is not difficult to see how readily mutations occur which give rise to a wide range of biological variants even within the same individual. These variants are called quasispecies. Many of the biological variations are of crucial importance to the pathogenesis of HIV infection and HIV disease, and the selection for variants which favours the progress of the virus in the body is the key to the ability of the virus to cause a progressive and ultimately fatal disease. Thus, over time the variants that develop are those associated with greater virulence and greater resistance to the body's defences. They are also responsible for the inevitable development of resistance of the virus to antiviral therapy, which occurs rapidly if the patient is treated with one drug only (Chapter 6).

One of the most important characteristics of variants are those related to the growth of the virus. Variants isolated from patients in the early silent phase of infection tend to be predominantly of the slow/low type; that is, they replicate slowly and, in cell cultures, have low yields of virus. As disease develops and progresses, the main variants isolated are the rapid/high type; that is, they replicate rapidly and have high yields of virus in cell culture. A further variation which relates to growth rate concerns their ability to produce syncytia in cell culture. Most authorities now recognize two groups of growth rate variants – low-replicating non-syncytium-inducing variants (often referred to as NSI variants) and the high-replicating syncytium-inducing variants (often referred to as SI variants), the latter correlating with the most advanced stages of the disease.

The range of cells that can be infected by each variant of HIV is also correlated with the stage of infection depending on which co-receptor is used for attachment. Thus, in the early silent stage of infection, HIV isolates are in the main able to infect predominantly the monocytes (called mono-cytotropic or macrophagetropic) (using the CCR-5 co-receptor). With advancing disease viral isolates develop an increasing ability to infect the lymphocytes (lymphotropic) (using the CXCR-4 co-receptor), and still later demonstrate a wider cellular host range and are able to infect a relatively large variety of cultured cells. The host range of HIV isolates varies not only with the stage of the disease, but also with the tissue or organs from which the virus was isolated. Thus, virus isolated from the blood and from the bowel have a wider host range than those from the brain. Other biological features are also dependent on the origin of the isolate; for example, isolates from the brain tend to be less virulent as measured by their cell-killing ability and more sensitive to neutralizing antibodies, than those from the blood.

Further biological variations which correlate with advancing disease and also greater virulence include: an increased affinity to attach to non-neutralizing antibodies and thus to promote antibody-mediated enhancement; a reduced sensitivity to the inhibitory effects of the protein encoded for by the *nef* gene (the negative regulatory protein of the virus, see Chapter 2, 'The AIDS virus – HIV' subsection 'The regulation of HIV'); and an increasing ability to disrupt and damage cell membranes.

The ability of HIV to evade the immune response of the host

Truly one of the most remarkable features of HIV infection is its un-paralleled ability to overcome the host's immune system. The inexorable progress of the illness in virtually all individuals who are infected, despite the presence of antibodies, has baffled scientists ever since the disease was first studied. A number of possibilities have been postulated as to how the virus is able to evade the immune system of the host. It was the detailed investigations of long-term non-progressors – those HIV-infected persons who remain healthy with good immune function for at least seven years after infection – which provided the first real answers to this enigma. The crucial component of the immune response to all virus infections, includ-ing HIV, is the CTLs, which destroy infected cells and inhibit viral repli-cation. In the initial stages of infection with HIV, the individual mounts a vigorous CTL response which is almost effective in removing the virus and sharply reduces the number of infectious virus particles. This immune response is responsible for producing the symptoms which are experienced by the patient in the acute disease stage. The large numbers of virus par-ticles present in the acute stage are cleared from the blood by the CTLs and, in the subsequent early silent phase, few or no virus particles are detectable in the blood. In this early stage of infection biochemical tests can demonstrate the presence of those cytokines produced by the CD4 lymphocytes which activate CTLs, i.e. a Th1 response. In the long-term non-progressors this Th1 cytokine profile is maintained for many years and these individuals therefore demonstrate a vigorous CTL response directed against HIV-infected cells; this is probably responsible for the ability of the host to resist the virus and keep down the viral numbers to a level where they do not cause disease. However, in the great majority of HIV-infected persons, the Th1 response of the CD4 lymphocytes is not maintained for very long and the cytokine profile switches to a Th2 pattern which activates, instead, the humoral arm of the immune system. Antibodies are therefore produced, but these are far less effective in neutralizing virus than are the CTLs. The virus numbers consequently build up, resulting in the progressive depletion of the CD4 lymphocyte population. Not only are the CD4 lymphocytes destroyed but those that remain are also damaged functionally, further reducing the capacity of the body to mount an effective CTL response.

Exactly what is responsible for the Th1 to Th2 switch is not clear, nor is it clear why the small minority of those infected with HIV, i.e. the long-term non-progressors, do not switch to a Th2 response, but maintain their effective anti-HIV CTL response for many years. The enormous variability of HIV may well play a role by placing an enormous strain on the functioning of the antigen-presenting cell, which is continuously called on to present new antigenic fragments for recognition by the CD4 lymphocytes. This ultimately exhausts the CD4 lymphocytes and destroys their functional capacity; or alternatively these stresses may stimulate the shift to a Th2 response. Antigenic variation may also be a mechanism by which the virus is able to escape detection by CTLs, as there is a finite repertoire of antigens which would be detected by CTLs on the surface of MHC I proteins on the target cells. Finally, HIV, like many other viruses which cause persistent infections, appears also to have evolved a mechanism of perturbing the process of antigen presentation by interfering with the antigen-presenting cell's ability to efficiently couple viral antigenic fragments onto the MHC II molecule.

Conclusion

HIV is a unique human pathogen. No other pathogen of humankind has evolved the variety of strategies that HIV has to evade the immune response of the host. Antigenic variability to avoid immune recognition, interrupting

JOHN MOORES UNIVERSITY AVRIL ROBARTS LRC TEL. 0151 231 4022 LIVERPOOL

the process of antigen presentation, interfering with CD4 helper lymphocyte function as well as destruction of CD4 lymphocytes are some of the
components of the onslaught on the immune system by HIV. These strategies have been so successful that, until recently, it appeared that once an
individual was infected it was inevitable that the virus would overcome
the immune system and ultimately cause a progressive and ultimately lethal
disease. While antiviral drugs have, to some extent, provided some renewed
optimism in being able to control HIV disease on a long-term or even permanent basis (Chapter 6), the immune system of the body may also hold
the key to addressing the control of HIV infection. Studies of long-term
non-progressors have provided new insights into the ability of the immune
system to successfully control HIV and they have also given scientists a
greater understanding of the strategies used by HIV to evade the immune
response. There are some important pieces of the puzzle which still need
to be completed. When these answers are forthcoming the therapeutic
manipulation of the immune system could add a further opportunity for
effectively controlling the infection by providing the means therapeutically to
maintain HIV-infected individuals in a permanent state of non-progression.

4

The transmission of HIV infection

The previous chapters have illustrated how truly extraordinary and unique the HIV virus is and how this remarkable virus is able to cause such a catastrophic disease by exploiting and capitalizing on a complex set of chinks in human immunological armour. However, there is nothing unusual or noteworthy about the transmissibility of this agent. In fact, in terms of its ability to transfer itself from one host to another, it ranks as one of the least efficient of viruses. Indeed, a number of the features of the virus and also the virus–host interaction, which are of such cardinal importance to the devastation that it causes, are distinct handicaps with respect to its transmissibility. Having the CD4 protein as a receptor site is a major factor in the profound depletion of CD4 lymphocytes but it also places severe limitations on the access sites in the body thatwhich are available to the virus. Being a highly variable virus is also highly advantageous firstly in enabling it to evade the host's immune response and subsequently in developing more virulent variants. At the same time, however, variability could be a relative handicap for the virus in that it imposes on it the because it means that requirement for a relatively large dose containing the spectrum of variants, for example, viruses which selectively infect the monocytes, which are is required for infection to be established in a new host; for example, this is the case for viruses that selectively infect the monocytes.

To become the successful infectious parasite of the body that HIV is, it has therefore had to adapt to a transmission route which minimizses its exposure to a hostile environment outside of the warm nurturing intracellular location in the human body. The venereal route is ideally suited for this. It is small wonder that many (although by no means all), of the venereally spread infectious agents are also relatively delicate organisms that have exploited the protection of the venereal route of transmission and, in exchange, have sacrificed the potential of much greater contagiousness which the other more hostile routes of transmission such as airborne and gastro-intestinal spread could have offered. However, because HIV also persists in the bloodstream, as does hepatitis B virus, it may, in addition to the venereal route, also be spread in situations where blood is exchanged between individuals. Thus the regular modes of transmission of HIV – venereal and blood exchange – arise from these relatively stringent requirements on the virus to ensure its successful transmission. On the odd occasion a particular unfortunate set of circumstances may arise where sufficiently high doses of virus containing the necessary viral variants may be transferred to a susceptible host who has the requisite CD4-containing cells in an activated form waiting to receive them. These circumstances can only very rarely mimic those offered regularly by the venereal and blood exchange routes but may, on occasion, be responsible for the unusual or even freakish incidents of HIV transmission which are reported from time to time and which receive inordinate publicity because of the abject fear of AIDS. Unfortunately, it is these episodes which have generated the exaggerated fears and even hysteria about the so-called 'contagiousness' and also the so-called 'casual transmission' of HIV.

Mechanisms of transmission

Source of the virus

HIV, like the majority of human viruses, is derived exclusively from human sources, that is individuals who are infected with the virus and who actively secrete infectious virus. In the case of HIV, unlike any other virus, all individuals who are infected are potentially sources of infectious virus, and remain so for the rest of their lives. The degree of viraemia (that is the presence of virus in the bloodstream) does, however, fluctuate with much greater amounts of infectious virus, and also more virulent variants, being demonstrable in the early stages soon after infection and also in the later stages in advanced AIDS disease. The degrees of infectiousness would correspond to these phases of heightened viraemia.

Infectious HIV has been isolated from most body fluids – blood (the cellular elements as well as plasma), cerebrospinal fluid (the fluid bathing the central nervous system), tears, saliva, semen, vaginal secretions and breast milk, but not in urine or in faeces. However, it is only from blood, semen and vaginal fluid that the virus can be regularly isolated. Thus, although there have been reports by a number of laboratories of HIV isolates being obtained from these other body secretions and body fluids, most other centres have not been successful in duplicating them. The presence of infectious virus in these secretions is thus, at best, a rare event or, in some cases, excessively rare. For example, saliva is a hostile body fluid for HIV – not only is there great dilution but, in addition, a number of substances have been identified in saliva which will readily inactivate the virus. However, any body fluid or secretion which is contaminated by blood is far more likely to have significant amounts of infectious virus in it. In the case of semen and vaginal fluid, both secretions are rich in lymphocytes including CD4 lymphocytes, and also the genital mucous membranes are extensively supplied with Langerhans cells. These cells are the major presenters of foreign antigen to the immune system. They are, in addition, highly susceptible to infection with HIV as their surface is rich in CD4 receptor sites. They can therefore function as vehicles to transport HIV from peripheral mucous membranes centrally to the lymphoid tissue of the immune system.

Viral features affecting transmission

Because of the variability of the virus and the need for particular variants to be included in the infecting dose, a relatively large mass of virus is required for transmission to be successful. This could be achievable by the source material having a high concentration of virus, as might occur in sexual secretions and in blood from individuals in either the early or the terminal stages of infection. Transmission of infection could also occur after a single exposure even with a very small volume of infectious material provided that it contained a sufficiently high concentration of virus with the necessary spectrum of variants. Alternately, infection may be transmitted following a single exposure to a large volume of virus-containing material, as would occur in a contaminated blood transfusion. Successful transmission of virus may also take place following recurrent and repetitive exposure to the virus where cumulatively a large enough infective dose of virus could build up.

As with most enveloped viruses, HIV is a relatively delicate organism which is susceptible to drying, sunlight and the other hostile influences found outside of the body. All enveloped viruses have therefore exploited transmission routes and mechanisms which minimize their time of exposure to the outside environment. Thus, many respiratory-spread viruses such as influenza and measles, which are similarly labile, have acquired extraordinarily efficient mechanisms of attaching to their receptor sites in the mucous membrane of the upper respiratory tract and are therefore readily and rapidly transmitted from host to host. HIV, however, does not have the same privilege of a highly efficient attachment mechanism, nor are the cells it needs to get to as readily exposed as in the case of the respiratory tract. The only routes which could be available to it are virtually restricted to sexual intercourse and the exchanging of blood itself. HIV has therefore had to sacrifice efficiency of transmission for the privilege of having CD4 antigen as its chief receptor site.

Influenza is probably the most contagious of all organisms and causes explosive outbreaks with very rapid spread of infection and the same is true of measles in susceptible populations. In contrast to this, HIV is poorly transmissible and epidemics in susceptible populations develop relatively slowly with new cases of infection occurring gradually, but progressively, over a prolonged period of time.

One of the characteristics of the human retroviruses is their strong dependence on being located inside cells for transmission to take place. Being transported intracellularly provides them with shelter against the outside environment, but is also important in the initiation of infection by cell-to-cell fusion rather than by virus–cell fusion. Thus, the human retrovirus HTLV-I appears to be totally dependent on intracellular transport for successful transmission of infection. In the case of HIV, extracellular transmission of virus can undoubtedly take place as, for example, has occurred tragically in thousands of haemophiliacs and other patients with bleeding disorders, who have been treated with cell-free clotting factor preparations derived from contaminated blood. However, extracellular transmission of virus is considerably less efficient and requires much higher doses of virus than intracellular transmission. It is probable that transmission involving relatively smaller volumes of material, as in the case of sexual transmission, depends on intracellular virus.

Access to the body

Although cells which do not contain CD4 receptors can be infected with HIV in the laboratory, present scientific evidence would suggest that transmission of infection in nature and the initial infectious episode areis dependent on the CD4 receptor site in addition to the co-receptor specific for macrophages or lymphocytes (Chapter 3). In other words, successful transmission of infection can only occur if HIV encounters CD4-bearing cells. Such cells are, of course, in abundance in the blood in the form of CD4 lymphocytes and monocytes. In addition, suitably susceptible CD4-bearing Langerhans cells are present in the mucous membranes of the body and are abundant in male and female genitalia.

In the rectal mucosa is found a specialized cell called the M-cell whose function is to transport foreign material, including viruses, across the rectal epithelial layer. The M-cell is closely associated with the lymphoid tissue found in the lining of the rectum and rapid transepithelial transport to lymphoid tissue and lymphocytes may well be part of the physiological immune response to foreign material entering the body via the bowel. M-cells could clearly also be an important portal of entry for HIV during rectal intercourse.

Due to the superficial presence both of Langerhans cells and M-cells, virus attachment and infection can occur through intact genital and rectal mucous membrane and it is not necessary to postulate that breaks or lacerations are obligatory for transmission to take place. However, it is also clear from numerous observations and studies, that infection occurs far more readily and more frequently when there is damage to genital or rectal mucosa, either through trauma or through ulcerating disease.

Langerhans cells are not restricted to the genitalia but are also present in other superficial mucous membranes of the body; for example, in the mouth and also in the skin. However, transmission of HIV cannot readily occur via the intact oral mucous membrane because of the dilution factor and also because of the presence of a number of antiviral materials in saliva which rapidly inactivate the virus. If sufficient virus were to be introduced through abrasions or lesions in the oral mucous membrane, infection could theoretically be transmitted via this route, although this has not been proven to occur in nature. Intact skin, however, forms a barrier which is impervious to infection with all viruses, not only HIV, as it is covered by a layer of dead keratin material called the stratum corneum (Fig. 4.1). As viruses are unable to propel themselves and are also unable to digest or penetrate through keratin should they land on intact skin, they would be unable to cross to living cells on which they depend in order to establish infection. However, if virus were to be introduced through the skin into the tissues below the keratin, for example as the result of a penetrating injury by a needle or sharp instrument, it would, of course, have access to the underlying susceptible Langerhans cells as well as blood cells.

The access points of HIV to the body are thus very limited and this, together with the substantive dosage requirements and the virus' lability, severely compromise the infectivity capabilities of HIV and also markedly restrict its routes of transmission.

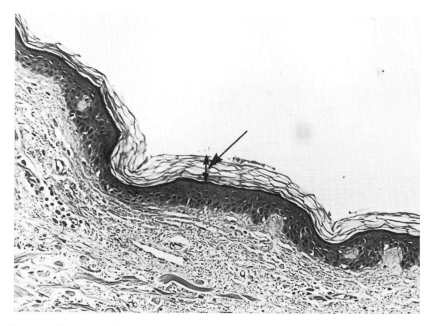

Fig. 4.1 Skin seen under the microscope (magnification 200×). Note the impervious barrier of keratin covering (arrowed) and protecting the skin cells.

Sexual transmission of HIV

Homosexual transmission

Since its earliest days, the AIDS epidemic in developed countries has been dominated by homosexual men and their lifestyle practices. In the majority of Western pattern 1 countries homosexual men still provide the bulk of AIDS cases – in the United Kingdom close on 90% of all reported AIDS cases occur in sexually active male homosexual or bisexual men.

It was also noted early on in the AIDS epidemic that rectal intercourse, specifically, was a high risk activity likely to promote the transmission of HIV. In particular, the receptive partner was especially in danger of acquiring infection because of the high frequency of trauma to the mucosal lining of the rectum during rectal intercourse. The rectal mucosa is a relatively delicate and friable epithelium composed of a lining of one cell thickness (Fig. 4.2) in contrast to the multi-cell layered and relatively robust vaginal epithelium which is far better equipped to withstand the injuries which may take place during intercourse (Fig. 4.3). Furthermore, the rectal wall is richly supplied with lymphoid tissue which can provide a ready access for the virus to susceptible lymphocytes (Fig. 4.4). The vaginal wall, on

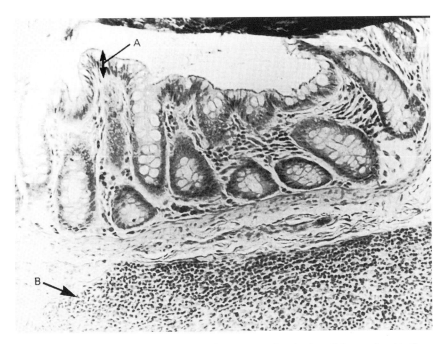

Fig. 4.2 Rectal mucous membrane which consists of a single-cell layered epithelium (A) with lymphoid tissue containing lymphocytes beneath it (B). (Magnification 200×.)

the other hand, has only sparse lymphoid tissue. Also the narrowness of the rectal canal makes it more vulnerable to trauma. Finally, the M-cells in the rectal mucosa are energetic transporters of foreign material to the underlying lymphoid tissue and lymphocytes. Clearly, the rectum is an organ which is far less adapted to sexual intercourse than the vagina and this puts it at especial risk for HIV infection.

There are, thus, a number of reasons to explain the special vulnerability of rectal intercourse to HIV infection, especially in comparison to vaginal intercourse. The rectal mucosa may also be damaged by other activities commonly practised by homosexual men, such as the insertion of the hand into the anus and rectum ('fisting') or the pushing of foreign objects, such as sex toys, into the rectum. Oro-genital and oro-anal ('rimming') contact is commonly practised by homosexuals but carries a very much smaller risk of infection.

Since the earliest days of the AIDS epidemic, sexual promiscuity was alleged to be a major factor in the rapid spread of HIV infection in the male homosexual community. Undoubtedly the profligate sexual trafficking and

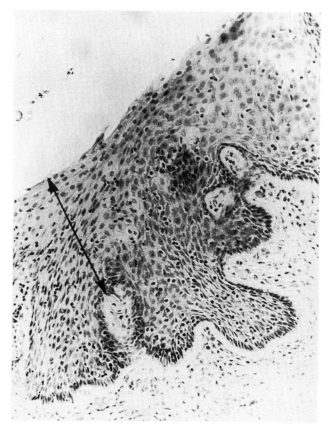

Fig. 4.3 Vaginal mucous membrane consisting of a robust multi-cell layered epithelium (arrowed). (Magnification 200×.)

indiscriminate sexual exchanges which were part of the culture of the bathhouses and other similar institutions were a significant component of the homosexual lifestyle in certain communities and this contributed very significantly to the rapid spread of HIV.

Female homosexuality or lesbianism has, on the other hand, played almost no role in the epidemiology of AIDS. Although penetrative sexual activities are practised by lesbians and the use of objects such as dildoes and other sex toys may cause vaginal trauma, there are virtually no opportunities in lesbian sexual activities for the exchange of substantial amounts of genital secretions. A few, almost freakish, incidents of HIV transmission between lesbians as a result of oro-genital contact have been reported. However, infections in lesbians have been due to heterosexual contact,

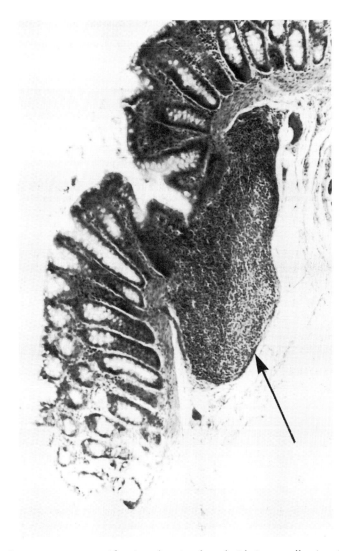

Fig. 4.4 Lower power magnification showing lymphoid tissue collection (arrowed) immediately underneath the rectal epithelium.

intravenous drug abuse and, in some cases, infection has been acquired from artificial insemination with semen which was obtained from high-risk homosexual male donors. Nevertheless the incidence of HIV infection in lesbians who are exclusively homosexual, who are not intravenous drug abusers and who have not been artificially inseminated is very much lower than for homosexual men.

Heterosexual transmission

Worldwide, heterosexual intercourse is the most common manner in which HIV is transmitted, even though in Western countries, such as the USA, it was implicated in only 13% of all reported cases of AIDS from 1993 to 1995 (although heterosexual transmission appears to be steadily increasing in Western countries). Initially it was postulated that breaches in the integrity of the vaginal or penile epithelium were essential for transmission to take place, even if these were only due to microscopic abrasions or lesions, as commonly does occur during sexual intercourse. However, the demonstration of the importance of Langerhans cells as the receptor cell for HIV infection and their abundance in the genital mucosa has now established how the virus could be transmitted through intact mucous membrane. Transmission through intact vaginal mucosa has been accomplished experimentally in monkeys with SIV and also observations of infections in women resulting from artificial insemination have added further confirmation of transmission through intact mucosa.

Nevertheless, as in the case of rectal intercourse, trauma to the vagina significantly increases the chances of transmission of HIV. Traumatic disruption of the vaginal mucosa is commonly seen in rape, which has resulted in a number of tragic cases of HIV infection, and also following the insertion of sex toys and other foreign objects into the vagina. Mucosal disruption due to ulcerating sexually transmitted diseases is a major co-factor for HIV transmission in the developing world, as will be discussed below. In the male, disruption of the epithelial integrity of the penis due to trauma or disease would similarly facilitate transmission of HIV.

In the absence of other co-factors, the transmissibility of HIV is far greater in the direction of male–female compared to female–male, in some studies of the order of twice as great and in others up to ten or more times as great. Considered mechanistically, this difference in transmissibility is not surprising. The female is, theoretically, considerably more vulnerable to infection because her vagina is a receptacle for a relatively large volume of infected semen, which then remains in contact with a substantial area of susceptible vaginal and cervical epithelium for prolonged periods of time. In contrast to this, the exposure of a susceptible male to an infected female involves only a brief contact with an infected epithelial surface and the retention of a thin film of vaginal or cervical secretion onto the susceptible epithelial surfaces of the penis and the urethra.

Oral sex and non-genital sex

There is little doubt that oral sex is vastly less likely to transmit infection than penile–vaginal or penile–anal sex. A few documented cases of HIV transmission via oral sex have been recorded, for example in impotent men who have practised only oral sex with prostitutes. On basic principles it could be deduced that the practice of fellatio (oro–penile sex) would carry a significantly greater risk than cunnilingus (oro–vaginal sex) because of the deposition of semen in the oral cavity, especially if there were to be lesions or abrasions in the oral epithelium. No differences in risk between these two forms of oral sex have, however, been established in nature. Any virus present in swallowed semen would be rapidly inactivated in the stomach contents.

It is not known whether HIV is transmissible via oro–anal contact. HIV is not found in faeces and it has not been established that the anal epithelium (which is structurally quite different to the rectal mucosa) is susceptible to the virus.

It has also not yet been established whetherthat HIV is transmissible via kissing, including so-called 'deep kissing' or 'French kissing' which involves the exchange of saliva. The virus, as mentioned previously, has on rare occasions been isolated from saliva, and, more recently, viral nucleic acid has been demonstrated by the highly sensitive polymerase chain reaction (PCR) technique in 50% of HIV-positive patients. The risk of transmission of virus would, of course, be substantially increased if infected blood is present in the saliva and, similarly, the susceptibility to infection would be increased if there were to be abrasions or lesions in the mouth due to trauma or disease. For these reasons, exposure to an infected person by deep kissing with salivary exchange is strongly discouraged even though actual transmission by this route has not as yet been definitively established to have occurred in nature.

Co-factors for sexual HIV transmission

The term 'co-factors' is used to describe biological factors which promote or facilitate the transmission of HIV or enhance the susceptibility of individuals to infection. The influence of co-factors in the development and progression of the HIV epidemic is enormous, especially in the developing world and in high-risk groups in the developed world. Their importance can be gauged by the vast difference in the heterosexually spread epidemics in developing and developed countries. In the developed world heterosexual transmission in the absence of co-factors is markedly less common than would be expected. For example, in studies of couples with an HIV-infected haemophiliac male partner it has been observed that only some 10–30% of their long-term female sexual partners (usually wives) become infected, in spite of the fact that few of these couples have regularly used condoms. In addition, the much greater likelihood of male–female transmission compared to female–male transmission is mainly seen in the absence of the effects of co-factors. In the developing world, where co-factors such as other sexually transmitted diseases are common, the frequency of female–male transmission is nearly the same as male–female. Finally, the mere fact that the HIV epidemic has not expanded to any major extent in the heterosexual population of Western countries to anything approaching the African situation, and is still only responsible for a relatively small percentage of AIDS cases, is powerful testimony of the influence that co-factors have in the transmission of the virus.

In contrast to this, in the developing world where HIV has cut a swathe of death and destruction, heterosexual intercourse is the overwhelming form of spread of AIDS in adults. While the risk of transmission of the virus is also directly proportional to the number and frequency of change of sexual partners, which does play a major role, undoubtedly biological co-factors – especially other sexually transmitted diseases and chronic diseases, particularly tuberculosis – play a cardinal role in the HIV epidemic in pattern 2 countries of the developing world.

Sexually transmitted diseases are a common cause of debility and even death in the developing world. These diseases are due to a variety of micro-organisms – viruses, bacteria, fungi and parasites. Clinically, sexually transmitted diseases present in three basic ways. Firstly, as ulcerative disease where the major clinical feature is the formation of ulcers on the genitalia which may or may not be painful and which may also be associated with varying degrees of associated lymph gland swelling; secondly, as genital discharge, usually with pain on urination; and thirdly, a miscellany of presentations specific to the causal organism, for example genital warts (or condyloma) caused by the wart virus and lymph gland swelling in the groin – also called inguinal buboes, etc. Of these, genital ulcer disease is the most important co-factor for HIV infection.

In Africa the most common cause of genital ulceration is a bacterium called *Haemophilus ducrei*, which causes a painful ulcer commonly referred to as soft chancre or chancroid (the term 'chancre' classically refers to the hard, painless genital ulcer found with syphilis soon after infection) (Figs. 4.5 and 4.6). This organism is susceptible to a number of antibiotics (although not penicillin) and is generally quite easily treated. Other causes

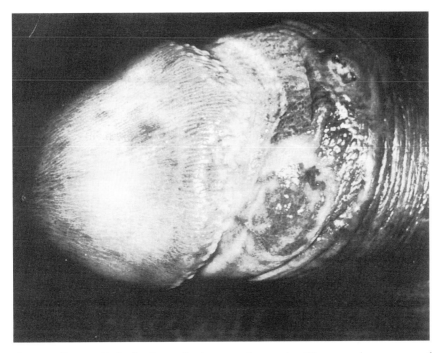

Fig 4.5 Chancroid (soft chancre) ulcer on the penis. (Photograph courtesy of Professor R C Ballard.)

of genital ulcer disease include syphilis (which is still relatively important in most of Africa in spite of it being readily treated with penicillin), and herpes simplex or genital herpes (which is the most common cause of genital ulcer disease in the developed world). The breach in the integrity of the genital mucosa from ulceration is an obvious mechanism for enhancing susceptibility to infection by allowing the virus ready access to lymphocytes and monocytes in the bloodstream. In addition, the associated inflammatory response attracts monocytes and macrophages and the immune response activates lymphocytes which further increases the vulnerability of the new host to HIV infection. Genital ulcers, especially in the case of chancroid, are friable lesions which bleed readily during sexual intercourse (the frequency of intercourse is rarely diminished by the pain of the lesion) and thus the chances of transmission of infection are also enhanced (Fig. 4.7).

Sexually transmitted diseases characterized by genital discharge also play an important role as co-factors for HIV transmission, particularly infection with a tiny bacterium called *Chlamydia trachomatis*. This organism is the most important agent responsible for the disease of non-gonococcal

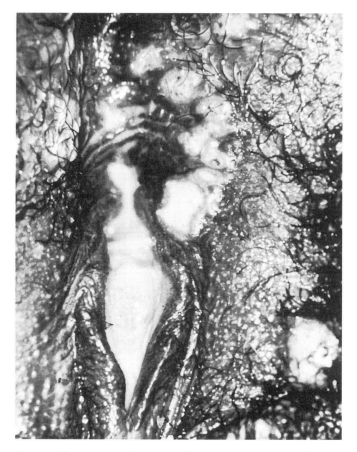

Fig. 4.6 Chancroid ulcers on the vulva. (Photograph courtesy of Professor R C Ballard.)

urethritis, often abbreviated to NGU (also referred to as non-specific urethritis or NSU) (Fig. 4.8). The classic cause of inflammation of the urethra and discharge is the gonococcus bacterium which caused gonorrhoea (colloquially referred to as 'the drop'). With the advent and the widespread use of penicillin, to which the organism is sensitive, gonorrhoea has to a large extent been replaced by infections with other, penicillin-resistant, organisms as causes of genital discharge and urethritis, hence the clinical entity of non-gonococcal urethritis. Chlamydial infection of the genital tract enhances susceptibility to infection by promoting the secretion of inflammatory cells into the genitalia including susceptible lymphocytes and especially monocytes. It also increases the friability of the cervix, often resulting

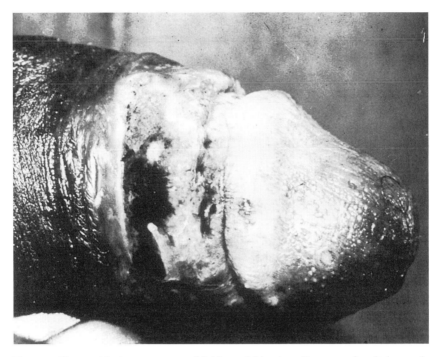

Fig. 4.7 Chancroid ulcers are very friable and bleed easily even after light swabbing to take a specimen. (Photograph courtesy of Professor R C Ballard.)

in the formation of tiny ulcers on the cervical epithelium and, in addition, induces 'ectopy of the cervix'. The term ectopy of the cervix (also referred to as 'cervical ectropion') is used to describe the outward movement of the epithelium from the canal of the cervix to the exterior of the cervix which lies within the vagina. The epithelium of the inner canal of the cervix (endo-cervix) is composed of a single layer of tall rectangular cells and is quite different in structure from the multi-layered, flattened epithelium found on the outer part of the cervix protruding into the vagina (ectocervix). This migration of endocervical epithelium to occupy an ectocervical location is commonly found in adolescents and is also associated with the use of the oral contraceptive pill and pregnancy. The consequent exposure of this sensitive epithelium to semen is thought to enhance susceptibility to HIV infection.

Another major co-factor promoting HIV transmission in developing countries is chronic generalized infections which are so prevalent especially in the tropics. Chronic tropical diseases, especially parasitic diseases, are responsible for a major proportion of illness, debility and death on the

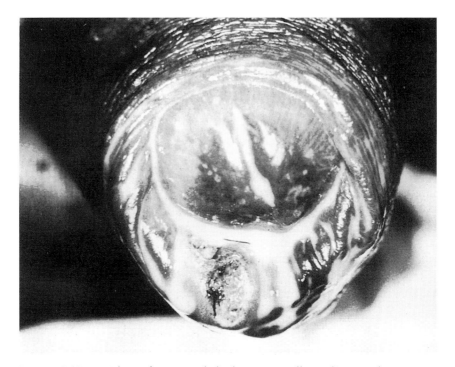

Fig 4.8 Patient with profuse genital discharge as well as ulcer on the prepuce. (Photograph courtesy of Professor R C Ballard.)

African continent and have now assumed an even greater importance because of the HIV epidemic. The resultant chronic activation and stimulation of lymphocytes may well be the mechanism for the enhanced susceptibility to HIV. In addition, many of these chronic illnesses are themselves associated with immunosuppression which may handicap the host's ability to respond to the initial HIV infection.

Malaria, one of the commonest infectious diseases of humankind and a major cause of death in Africa, was one of the first of the tropical diseases to be implicated as a co-factor for HIV. Indeed, in earlier scientific literature, virtually all malaria patients tested for HIV were positive. Later, however, it was shown that the HIV antigen and those of the malaria antigens are so similar that they cross-react (in other words, they will react positively in each other's tests) and malaria antigens could give a false-positive test for HIV. More recent studies have found that malaria is not an important co-factor in HIV transmission.

Worldwide, the most important chronic infection to be associated with

HIV infection is tuberculosis. Today, tuberculosis still remains as one of the major diseases of humans – approximately one-third of the human population is infected. The WHO has estimated that there are eight to ten million new cases of tuberculosis each year in the world and two to three million deaths, over three-quarters of these in tropical countries. In sub-Saharan countries up to one-half of the adult population has been infected.

In developed countries there has been a serious resurgence of tuberculosis, especially in deprived inner-city populations. Thus, in the USA, the declining incidence was halted in the mid-1980s and is now again on the increase, due primarily to the HIV epidemic. Tuberculosis, as with other chronic infectious diseases, enhances susceptibility to HIV infection because of lymphocyte activation and immunosuppression. Conversely, the immunosuppression of HIV infection enhances susceptibility to infection with the tuberculosis bacterium and it also activates latent tuberculosis in individuals who have previously been infected. (The tuberculosis organism, as in the case of HIV, tends to remain latent or dormant in the body after the initial primary infection and may be activated later in life by various triggering factors.) Tuberculosis has, therefore, now become the most important opportunistic infection in AIDS in developing countries. The problem is becoming even further compounded by the increasing occurrence of tuberculosis caused by organisms which are resistant to most of the antibiotics and drugs used in its treatment.

A further important co-factor in HIV transmission, particularly seen in developing countries, is the absence of male circumcision. It has been observed in a number of studies that uncircumcised males are significantly more susceptible to HIV infection than those who are circumcised. The enhanced susceptibility of the uncircumcised state is probably due to the frequent presence of infection in the foreskin and the glans penis, the greater chance of trauma to the foreskin, maceration of the skin of the penis and also the more prolonged contact with HIV-infected material trapped in the foreskin.

The oral contraceptive pill has also been shown to enhance susceptibility to infection. This is probably related to the effect of the oestrogen hormone component of the pill, which causes ectopy of the cervix and also may be responsible for some degree of immunosuppression and to some extent increases the risk of chlamydial infection, which is itself a co-factor for HIV infection.

The relationship between sexual intercourse during the menstrual period and enhanced female–male transmission has been investigated in a number of studies. On theoretical grounds contact with infected blood including lymphocytes and monocytes should facilitate transmission of HIV to the male partner. However, this has not as yet been verified.

The use of so-called 'recreational drugs' such as cocaine and cannabis, which are frequently partaken together with sexual activity, may well also enhance susceptibility to infection because of their immunosuppressive effects. Similarly nitrites, which are often used by homosexual men to promote and prolong erection, have marked immunosuppressive activities.

Prevention of sexual transmission

The options for the prevention of HIV transmission during sexual intercourse are, of course, a major component of the educational efforts to promote safer sexual practices. Foremost amongst these options is the condom (Fig. 4.9). There is little doubt that, when correctly used, the condom is a highly effective barrier which is very successful in preventing the transmission of all sexually transmitted diseases, including HIV. Nevertheless, failures do occur. The breakage rate of latex condoms during vaginal intercourse has been variously estimated to be up to 13%, while in rectal intercourse

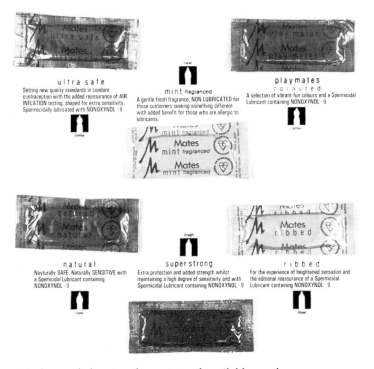

Fig 4.9 Display card showing the variety of available condoms.

these same condoms may break up to 50% of times. This has prompted some condom manufacturers to produce more robust condoms for rectal use. Precisely how effective condoms are in preventing HIV infection is difficult to determine. The failure rate of condom usage for contracept has been estimated at up to 13–15%. Analysis of these failures implic user failure to a far greater extent than product failure. There are a num of causes of condom user failure. Examples are: putting the condom o too late a stage of intercourse, that is, after some ejaculation has alre taken place; leaving an inadequate space in the reservoir of the condom to collect semen, which may cause it to burst; removal of the condom too late causing it to slip off when the penis is flaccid and spilling the semi-nal contents into the vagina; tearing of the condom by sharp fingernails and rings. These are all some of the more common causes of user error and condom failure. Product failure may be the result of the condom being too old or having been incorrectly stored; for example, in hot conditions or in sunlight, or due to it being re-used or being used with an oil-based lubricant, which destroys rubber, instead of a recommended water-based lubricant. Condoms obtained from reputable manufacturers are tested for strength (Fig. 4.10) and should bear a national quality mark.

More recently a female condom, also called a Femidom, has been devel-oped. It is also manufactured from latex rubber and is inserted into the vagina to cover the entire vaginal and cervical surface with its uppermost ring sitting outside the vagina on the pubis. The intrusiveness of this device has been a drawback and there have thus been reservations expressed as to its acceptability. It does, however, provide the woman with a means of controlling her own sexual health. The efficacy of the Femidom is currently under evaluation.

A number of spermicidal substances used in contraception, as well as antiseptic materials used in sexual hygiene, have been examined for their activity against HIV. Foremost amongst these is a compound called nonoxynol-9, which is the active ingredient in a number of widely used spermicide contraceptives. It has been shown to have potent activity against HIV and is now commonly incorporated into pre-lubricated condoms. The efficacy of nonoxynol-9-containing lubricant jellies or sponges on their own for preventing HIV infection is, however, doubtful as they would need to be in contact with the virus for at least a number of seconds for it to be effective, and infected semen may well bypass any meaningful contact time with themit. It has also been advocated that nonoxynol-9 should to be included in vaginal douches or rectal enemas after, for example, rape by a suspected infected assailant. However, the trauma of the douche or enema

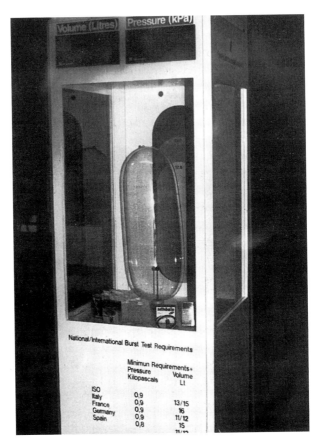

Fig 4.10 Apparatus to text condom strength.

may itself inadvertently enhance HIV infection and these post-exposure procedures are now no longer recommended.

An indirect but extremely important option for preventing sexual HIV transmission is the addressing of the problem of sexually transmitted diseases. Clearly, the treatment of these diseases, especially genital ulcer disease, would in itself be an important means of preventing HIV transmission.

HIV transmission by blood exchange

Blood transfusion

The acquisition of HIV infection by blood transfusion or products derived from blood has always elicited particular sympathy and compassion from the general public. Fortunately, in developed countries and in many developing countries, the incidence of transfusion-acquired HIV infection has dropped dramatically and it is now a relatively rare route of transmission. This is due solely to the success of prevention measures and, at present, it is only this transmission route where options for prevention have been really effective.

The direct infusion of a large volume of infected blood containing millions of infected cells into the bloodstream of another person would, one would expect, result in the universal transmission of infection. However, studies have shown that although the transmission rate for blood transfusion is by far the highest for any route of transmission, over 90% of recipients of infected blood become infected, there does remain, nevertheless, a small percentage of individuals who appear to be resistant to infection. These individuals are, of course, extremely valuable in attempts to elucidate the mechanisms of resistance to HIV infection. The blood transfusion route, being by far the most effective route of transmission, would provide the best model to study this resistance. Theoretically, failure of infection (after blood transfusion) could be due to the occurrence of an unusually fortunate circumstance of a very low level of virus in the blood of the seropositive donor. However, given the enormous volume of infected material which is transferred, this would be highly unlikely. As discussed in Chapter 3, certain individuals may genetically be resistant to infection with HIV because of mutations in the CCR-5 co-receptor required by HIV to infect macrophages.

Blood products

While blood obtained from donors may be used therapeutically as whole blood, frequently it is the various components of blood which are extracted and utilized clinically. For example the plasma (i.e. the fluid portion of blood which remains after the cells have been removed) or alternately the cells alone (often referred to as 'packed cells') may be administered therapeutically. In some cases only certain cells are used, for example the white cells or platelets, for treating different medical conditions. Proteins extracted from the plasma are also frequently used clinically; for example, immunoglobulins (the proteins of which antibodies are composed) are used to give immediate (albeit temporary) protection to individuals exposed to certain infectious diseases (passive immunization). Individuals with bleeding disorders such as haemophilia are treated with proteins which promote the clotting of blood, called clotting factor or factor VIII in the case of haemophilia, or other factors with some of the other bleeding disorders.

These various components and protein fractions carry different risks of transmission of HIV. Theoretically blood products containing infected lymphocytes and monocytes would be assumed to be the most infectious. Thus, packed cells would carry, theoretically, as great a risk as whole blood. Nevertheless it is known that HIV can be transmitted if the virus is outside the cells, that is in the plasma, although a larger dose would be needed. Of the plasma protein fractions, certain are more likely to contain virus than others. In particular, clotting factor is especially rich in a number of viruses including HIV because the process of extraction and concentration of this protein also has the effect of concentrating many viruses of similar molecular size and mass. However, proteins such as immunoglobulins are molecularly quite different from viruses and in the concentration and purification process these proteins become freed from any contaminating viruses in the blood. Thus, immunoglobulin preparations used for passive immunization are safe and do not carry a major risk of HIV infection.

Needle and syringe sharing

In Western countries with pattern 1 AIDS, the second largest group of AIDS patients after the homosexual male group is that of the intravenous drug abuser, that is individuals who habitually inject drugs into their veins and share syringes and needles or re-use them without adequate sterilization. In the USA intravenous drug abuse is responsible for some one-third of all AIDS cases and in some European countries it comprises the largest single group of AIDS patients; for example, in Italy and Spain over 50% of AIDS patients are intravenous drug abusers. Frequently intravenous drug abuse is also associated with other high risk behaviour such as sexual promiscuity, for example prostitution, to sell sexual favours for drugs.

The HIV epidemic in the intravenous drug abusing population has often been characterized by very rapid spread and high prevalences of infection. Viral transmission is facilitated by three features in this population. First of all, there is the repetitiveness of needle-sharing experiences and the exchanging of not insubstantial volumes of blood. The sharing of needles and syringes is itself part of the culture, for example in the so-called 'shooting galleries', where illicit drugs are mixed with blood in the barrel of the syringe and shared between participants. Even in seemingly empty syringes, a reasonable volume of blood may remain behind as a film between the barrel and the plunger of the syringe and also inside the hollow-bore needle. In simulated experiments this volume has been estimated to vary from 18–67 microlitres or μl (that is 0.018–0.067 ml). Even in the absence of deliberate sharing, the re-use of syringes and needles that have not been sterilized, or inadequately sterilized, is common in the world of illicit drug use.

A second factor promoting HIV transmission amongst intravenous drug abusers is the frequency of co-factors. The majority of these individuals are infected with viruses such as hepatitis B virus and cytomegalovirus as well as a number of bacterial and fungal infections. The drugs themselves are immunosuppressive and enhance susceptibility to infection and, in addition, sexually transmitted diseases are common.

Thirdly, as it is a criminal offence in most countries of the world to possess and to use these drugs and in many of these countries offences are subject to severe punishment, this group is the most marginalized and inaccessible of all the high-risk groups to any educational efforts. Programmes to supply needle exchange depots to furnish sterile needles and syringes in exchange for used ones have been controversially received, as they do give official recognition to a criminal offence. Educational messages regarding the proper sterilization of needles and other paraphernalia are often only able to reach their targets with difficulty. As a result there has been relatively little impact in slowing down the spread of HIV infection amongst intravenous drug abusers.

Injuries by needles and sharp instruments

The threat of HIV infection by the accidental inoculation of infected blood through penetrating injuries with needles or sharp instruments, so-called needle-stick injuries, has become one of the most contentious and emotive issues in the ethics of the practice of medicine and its allied professions. The fear of contracting HIV infection from a patient has sometimes assumed panic proportions and has materially affected the career choices of many young people, either within the specialities of the profession or even to enter the profession itself. It has given rise to unfair ostracism and discrimination against HIV-infected patients and, in some cases, compromised the quality of medical care. No less has The fear of needle-stick-acquired HIV infection in the medical profession has also affected the behaviour of the person in the street, in andfor example his relationship to his barber, or to hers to her beautician using electrolysis, let alone the totally groundless fears of the toilet seat and the door handle.

There is undoubtedly a finite risk of acquiring HIV infection by accidental needle-stick injury. In prospective investigations, that is following up, over years, health care workers who have sustained such injuries to see whether they become infected, some 73 such professionals have to date (1995) been documented worldwide to have become infected. In retrospective studies, that is investigating the past histories of health care workers who are HIV positive, in 141 such cases it was believed that infection was acquired through their work as a result of an injury with needles or instruments contaminated with infected blood from a patient. In contrast to this, hepatitis B virus, which is similarly transmitted, accounts for some 12 000 infections in physicians in the USA per year. Thus, even though the mortality from hepatitis B is only about 1% that of HIV, it is still responsible for far more occupationally acquired deaths. The risk of acquiring HIV infection from a deep penetrating injury with a needle contaminated with HIV-infected blood has been estimated to be of the order of 0.3%; that is, for every 300 such injuries one infection could result. Clearly this figure is a very approximate one. The risk for a more superficial injury is very much smaller. The risk also varies greatly with the stage of infection in the patient whose blood contaminated the needle as well as the susceptibility, in terms of co-factors, of the individual who has been pricked. In practice the risk must be very small indeed. Surgeons, gynaecologists and related professionals regularly inflict injuries on themselves with needles or scalpels which are contaminated with patients' blood. Over a lifetime the average surgeon would have sustained many hundreds of such injuries. Nevertheless, the incidence of AIDS in the health care professions is no higher than in the rest of the population. Thus, in the USA, the 5.4% of all AIDS cases which occurred in health care workers (as at 1988) was similar to the figure of 5.7% which is the proportion of the total labour force involved in the health care professions. Yet despite all this rational and logical reassurance fear persists. Undoubtedly precautions to protect health care workers from being exposed to needle-stick injuries must be energetically implemented and rigorously enforced, but exaggerated fears should not compromise the health care needs of infected patients.

The precise mechanism of transmission of infection via the needle-stick route has not definitively been established. In contrast to the needle-share transfer of infection that occurs in intravenous drug abusers, in accidental needle-stick incidents the volume of infected blood transferred is some 10 to 1000 times less if a contaminated hollow-bore needle inflicts the injury. The volume of contaminated blood would be considerably smaller even than this if the injury was due to a solid needle (such as a suturing needle) or a solid instrument (such as a scalpel blade).

Prevention of infection by the blood exchange route

To date, the most successful single achievement in the prevention of HIV infection has been the drastic reduction in transfusion-acquired infection resulting mainly from effective screening of donated blood. Throughout the developed world and in much, although by no means all, of the developing world donated blood is routinely screened by serological tests for the presence of antibodies. The diagnostic test which is mainly used is the ELISA (enzyme-linked immunosorbent assay) test (discussed more fully in Chapter 5). Such have been the advances in the diagnostic technology of HIV infection that today the ELISA test for the detection of HIV antibodies is perhaps the most exquisitely sensitive of all viral serological tests (of the order of 99.7%). This would mean that about three in every 1000 positive blood specimens screened would not be detected by the test and could possibly slip through and be utilized for transfusion.

In addition to the technological inadequacy of the test itself, a further difficulty in the screening of blood for HIV infection is the absence of antibodies in individuals shortly after infection, the so-called 'window period'. This period extends from the time the individual is first infected until the development of detectable antibodies. This early phase of infection which, although it is invisible to laboratory screening procedures, is nevertheless a stage of high infectivity with large amounts of virus in the blood and usually lasts for six to eight weeks, although in exceptional circumstances may stretch to many months or even sometimes up to a few years. On average a blood specimen in the 'window period' is encountered once in every 1000 positive blood specimens.

However, the actual risk of acquiring HIV infection from donated blood which has been screened is many orders of magnitude less than one in a thousand. The true risk can be calculated by multiplying the risk of an infected individual donating blood (that is the prevalence of HIV in the population of prospective blood donors) by the risk of positive blood not being detected because of shortcomings in the screening procedures. The prevalence of HIV in a population of prospective blood donors is considerably less than in the general population because voluntary blood donors are often the more socially responsible segment of society and are less likely to be infected with HIV (paid blood donors are being phased out throughout the world and are being replaced by voluntary blood donors). In addition, an important component of the efforts of blood banks to prevent transfusion of transmitted HIV is to actively discourage individuals in high risk categories, such as sexually active homosexual men, from d blood. The usual prevalence of HIV in such a population of blood donors in a pattern 1 Western country would be les some countries even 10 to 100 times less). Thus, the acquiring infection from a blood transfusion cor' approximately 0.0001% (0.1% × 0.1%), that million per unit of blood. Therefore, a blood ba.

units of blood per year could theoretically expect about ten transfusion-acquired HIV cases each year. This kind of risk has indeed been borne out in practice where new cases of transfusion-acquired HIV have now become a rarity since routine screening has been instituted.

Clearly, blood transfusion is still not a totally innocuous procedure despite the huge advances in diagnostic technology for HIV as well as other organisms, and also the success in reducing the number of high-risk individuals donating blood. Nevertheless, the risk of acquiring HIV infection has now become considerably less than that of a number of other infections and also less than other intrinsic risks of blood transfusion.

With regard to blood products, a great deal of research effort has been devoted to the development of techniques to treat blood and more especially blood products themselves, to inactivate any HIV virus which may be present. Pasteurization techniques, which involve heating to 60°C for 30 minutes, thus inactivating moderate doses of contaminating HIV, have been reasonably successful in treating clotting factor products. A number of chemical substances such as sorbitol or psoralen, which are effective in inactivating HIV while at the same time being relatively non-toxic, are also under evaluation.

The problem of HIV transmission in intravenous drug abusers has been one of the most taxing of the AIDS prevention challenges. The difficulties in accessing individuals who practise what is, in most countries, a criminal activity, has been alluded to above. Programmes for the exchange of dirty needles and syringes for clean sterile ones have been established in certain countries (Fig. 4.11), but have had the counter-effect of being a magnet, not only for drug addicts, but also drug dealers and criminal elements. The practice of the deliberate sharing of needles and syringes clearly needs to be urgently addressed. Where used needles and syringes cannot be replaced, sterilization procedures such as boiling, or the use of disinfectants such as bleach, need to be taught and promoted.

To prevent accidental injuries with needles or sharp instruments in the health care setting, most authorities have recommended and instituted policies of the so-called universal blood precautions. With this approach all patients who have to have procedures or operations performed on them must be handled and treated as if they were HIV infected and the appropriate precautions taken to prevent the occurrence of accidental penetrating injuries. There are large segments of the health care profession which insist on the routine screening of patients for HIV and then labelling positive patients so that extra care can be taken in handling them. Routine patient screening for HIV has generally been rejected for ethical reasons (to be

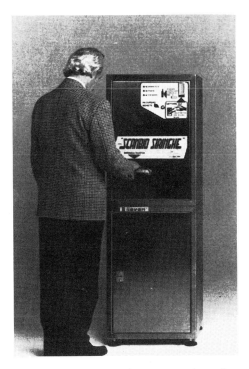

Fig 4.11 Advertising leaflet for automated syringe and needle exchange.

discussed in Chapter 8). Furthermore, as we have seen above, a small percentage of infected patients may still be missed on testing and these patients would pose an even greater danger to health care workers if they were to be treated in a more relaxed manner.

Many handbooks and guidelines for universal precautions have been published by various bodies. Essentially the elements of these precautions consist of ways of minimizing the risks of penetrating injuries such as avoiding the dangerous practice of replacing used needles into their plastic sheaths as these needles frequently slip and prick a finger. Used needles must be discarded into a puncture-resistant container which is then correctly disposed of (Fig. 4.12). Attempts should be made, where feasible, to modify surgical techniques to minimize the use of scalpels or suturing with needles (by using, for example, staples), or using needle holders to manipulate suturing needles. Reasonable protective clothing should be provided to prevent splashes of blood or other infected material onto the eyes or mouth. Blood spills on floors or tables need to be cleaned immediately and disinfected with an appropriate disinfectant such as bleach. If needle-stick or

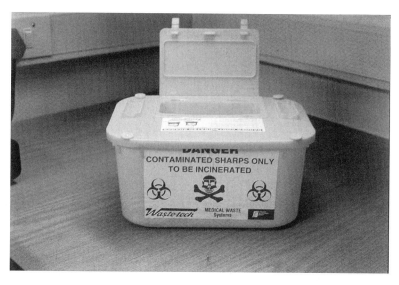

Fig. 4.12 Sharps disposal box for safe disposal of needles, blades and other sharp disposable items.

similar injuries do occur, they need to be reported immediately and the wound should be encouraged to bleed (to mechanically flush out any virus) without further traumatizing or squeezing the affected site, and it should also be gently washed with a disinfectant soap. Consideration may then need to be given whether to administer prophylactic anti-HIV drug therapy to prevent infection. This issue of post-exposure antiviral prophylaxis after accidental needle-stick injury will be dealt with more fully in Chapter 6.

Vertical transmission – mother-to-child

The most biologically intimate association between two individuals is that between a mother and the foetus developing in her womb. It is clear, therefore, that with such close contact of foetal tissues and maternal tissues over a fairly lengthy gestation period of nine months, the risk of transmission of HIV infection from mother to infant is second only to the risk of acquiring infection from a blood transfusion. Infection may be transmitted while the foetus is still in the uterus or during the delivery process as the infant moves down the birth canal and through the mother's genitalia and is bathed by the mother's blood during the birth process. Infection may also be acquired after birth by the baby ingesting milk from the mother. The transmission of infection from the mother to her child is referred to as vertical transmission. This route of transmission is by far the major route for paediatric infection (paediatric infection due to blood transfusion is now becoming increasingly uncommon because of routine screening). In developing countries, paediatric infection is now responsible for up to 15% of all AIDS cases. To date (1997) it has been estimated that some three million children have been infected – equivalent to 1000 babies being infected every day.

Mechanisms of vertical transmission

Infection may be transmitted while the foetus is still in the uterus (intrauterine or transplacental infection) or soon after birth (perinatal infection) and by breast feeding. Most transmission, 65%, occurs close to the time of delivery or during the birth process itself; 23% occurs *in utero* even as early as the first trimester and in only 12% of cases does transmission take place through breast feeding. The pathway of intrauterine transmission of virus from mother to child is not simply via the passive diffusion of virus from the mother's bloodstream to that of the foetus. Although there may well be some mixing of maternal and foetal blood through leaks or tears in the placenta, the latter generally forms a fairly effective barrier between the two bloodstreams. Infection of the infant in the uterus is, in fact, an active process where the placenta itself first needs to be infected, after which the virus may then spread to the infant.

In perinatal infection the infant is infected by contact with infected blood from the mother during birth, either through the infant's intact mucous membranes or through abrasions or lacerations which often occur during birth. With breast feeding the virus is assumed to enter through the infant's oral mucous membrane.

The risk of vertical transmission

The overall risk of transmission from an infected mother to her infant is approximately 30% but, as with other modes of transmission, there are wide variations. In pattern 1 developed countries the risk is considerably smaller; for example, European figures as low as 13% have been published, in contrast to those of up to 50% for Africa. The likelihood of transmission would also vary with the stage of HIV infection in the mother and consequently the level of virus in her blood (viral load). Thus, in the early stages of infection and also in the more advanced stages with severe immunosuppression, the risk of transmission to the infant is considerably higher. When the disease of AIDS itself occurs during pregnancy the majority of infants, up to 80%, would be at risk of infection. Various obstetric factors can increase the rate of transmission. For example, if the membranes have been ruptured for more than four hours before delivery takes place, procedures such as amniocentesis especially if they cause blood to enter the amniotic fluid, and premature labour, all significantly increase the rate of transmission. The presence of sexually transmitted disease and pelvic inflammatory disease during pregnancy also increases the risk of vertical transmission of HIV.

One of the most gratifying successes in the antiviral treatment of HIV has been the success in preventing vertical transmission of HIV by a short course of zidovudine during pregnancy. Initial clinical trials demonstrated a 70% reduction in transmission, irrespective of the viral load in the mother given a short course of zidovudine during pregnancy. This short course of therapy is still beyond the reach of most Third World countries where the need is most acute. Nevertheless, zidovudine treatment of pregnant mothers to prevent vertical transmission is the most significant therapeutic advance in the management or prevention of HIV infection to date.

Prevention of vertical transmission

The value of Caesarian section to reduce the likelihood of infection of the infant by avoiding the birth canal during delivery remains controversial. There have been studies which demonstrated a benefit and others have shown no difference in the rate of transmission. In the majority of countries of the world, HIV infection is sufficient grounds to legally abort a pregnancy. Routine antenatal screening of pregnant mothers for HIV infection, with the option of abortion if HIV positive, has been practised in a number of countries in an effort to reduce the growing number of paediatric HIV-infected cases.

The most widely accepted policy regarding breast feeding is that HIV-infected mothers should avoid breast feeding unless there is a danger of malnutrition in the infant as in socially deprived circumstances. In socio-economically poor communities the policy has been to recommend that HIV-infected mothers continue with breast feeding, because the risk of malnutrition often outweighs the lesser danger of HIV infection by breast feeding.

The relative risks of HIV transmission

Regular transmission routes of HIV

Each of the following routes of transmission plays an important role in the epidemiology of HIV. The route with the highest risk of HIV transmission is blood transfusion where the efficiency of transmission is over 90%, although it is now only responsible for fewer than 5% of all new HIV cases worldwide. The route with the second highest risk is vertical transmission which is responsible for up to 15% of all new HIV cases in pattern 2 countries and has a transmission rate of about 30%. Next, in terms of risk, is sexual intercourse. Rectal intercourse, especially for the receptive partner, carries a considerably greater risk than vaginal intercourse. In the latter, male–female transmission is significantly more efficient than female–male. When co-factors, especially genital ulcer disease, are present the efficiency of transmission, as discussed above, may be equal in both directions. The risk of sexual transmission does vary widely (and especially if co-factors are present or absent) but has been estimated at between less than 0.1 and 5.0% per sexual exposure. Vaginal intercourse is responsible for the bulk of new HIV cases worldwide, some 60–70%, and rectal intercourse approximately 5–10%. The sharing of needles by intravenous drug abusers carries a risk of about 0.5–1.0% per exposure, but again with wide variations, and is responsible for about 5–10% of all new HIV cases globally.

Rare transmission events

These rare incidents of HIV transmission which have been recorded have often engendered considerable anxiety and alarm, but are in fact of no meaningful consequence to the HIV epidemic. In this category could be included the transmission of HIV infection by needle-stick injury, of which not many cases have been recorded worldwide. In developed countries the odd cases of transfusion-acquired HIV infection could now also be included in this category.

Freak incidents and theoretical possibilities

A number of highly unusual incidents of HIV transmission have been reported in the scientific literature and have also often achieved exaggerated and often sensationalistic publicity in the mass media. In many cases the implications that have been deduced from these incidents have been exaggerated to the point of absurdity. Some of these incidents include a few recorded episodes of virus transmission through body contact sports such as boxing or, as was widely published, an incident where two football players collided with each other on the playing field resulting in bleeding injuries to both and transmission of infection took place, either due to the contact on collision or from the use of a communal sponge. A few incidents of transmission have been reported following fist fights, and in one case in an individual who habitually beat up homosexuals – 'gay bashing'. A similar odd incident occurred to an American on a visit to Rwanda in Central Africa, who was involved in a bus accident which resulted in him being pinned down by several bleeding passengers lying on top of him. He himself sustained multiple lacerations which, presumably, were the portal of entry for virus from one of the bleeding passengers lying on top of him.

In all of these freakish incidents, transmission of HIV was probably the result of an extremely unfortunate set of coincidences and a number of factors favouring the transmission of the virus. Successful transmission would have required a particularly high concentration of virus in a minute amount of blood, the presence of the correct of variant strains of virus, the transfer of a sufficient amount of this blood through breaks in the skin or mucosa to a recipient individual who was, in all probability, at a high level of susceptibility due to various co-factors including the presence of activated lymphocytes at the site of inoculation. This assemblage of cir- cumstances can clearly only occur on extremely rare occasions and does little to change the concept of HIV being an agent of particularly low trans- missibility which can only be infectious under very specific circumstances involving the intimate exchanging of body fluids either in substantial amounts or at regular repetitive intervals leading eventually to accumulation of a large enough dose of virus.

Various theoretical possibilities of HIV transmission have been postu- lated and have been carefully considered and rigorously researched. Perhaps the most widely publicized of these is that of insect transmission. It has been clearly established that needles which penetrate the skin are able to transmit infection as has been discussed above. In the case of needle- sharing, infection occurs at a relatively high level of efficiency, but infec- tion from needle-stick injuries only rarely occurs. It would thus seem to be a logical extension that human-biting and blood-sucking insects which are, in essence, flying syringes, could also be able to transmit infection. There is indeed a very important family of viruses that are mainly trans- mitted from human-human by biting arthropods (insects and ticks) and that affect both humans and animals. These viruses are called arboviruses and include those that cause such well known diseases as yellow fever and dengue. In the case of the arboviruses there is active multiplication of virus in the cells of the arthropod host before being inoculated into the human host. With HIV, however, there is no possibility that the virus can multiply in insect cells. There is considerable, albeit not conclusive, evidence that the hepatitis B virus, which shares the same routes of transmission as HIV

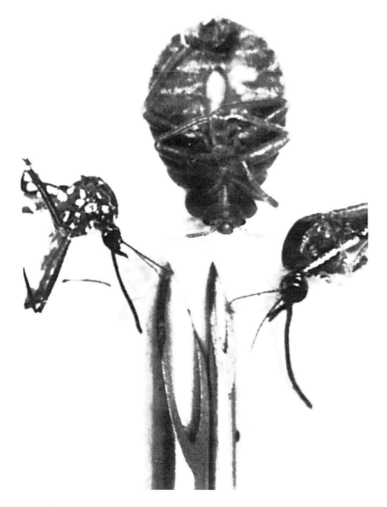

Fig. 4.13 Bed bug (top), mosquitoes (left and right) and needles (bottom) under the microscope (×50 magnification). The thicker needle (18G) is commonly used to take blood and the thinner needle (23G) is commonly used for administering injections.

and is also unable to multiply in insect cells, may nevertheless be mechanically transmitted by biting arthropods from person to person. Nevertheless, hepatitis B virus has been shown to be many orders of magnitude more infectious than HIV, and it has been calculated that the amount of blood which could be transported mechanically in the proboscis, or mouth parts, of an arthropod would be far too small for it to be able to mechanically transfer an adequate volume of blood in the case of HIV (Fig. 4.13). Epidemiologically, there is also absolutely no evidence that arthropod transmission plays any role whatsoever in HIV infection. There is, for example, no evidence that HIV infection is in any way more common in individuals who have been infected by other arthropod-borne viruses. Neither is there any evidence of HIV infection being associated with individuals living in ecological niches favourable either for arthropods or for the combination of arthropods and HIV. Thus, no true scientist can totally and categorically dismiss the remote possibility that arthropods could transmit HIV. However, what can be stated incontrovertibly is that if arthropods were to be able to transmit HIV, they could not have anything other than an exceedingly small role in its epidemiology.

Impossible transmission routes

With regard to some of the 'possibilities' which do surface from time to time, there is no way, even theoretically, by which HIV could be transmitted by these routes. For example by ingestion through the gastro-intestinal tract where the virus would be rapidly inactivated. There is also no way that infection could be acquired by inhaling the virus from the air unless, theoretically, in very highly concentrated aerosols generated in the laboratory setting. Virus present on inanimate objects such as toilet seats or door handles cannot transmit infection, as even were it to survive in a drop of organic material, it could not penetrate through intact skin. Similarly, HIV would not be able to survive for any significant period of time on the intact skin of a patient with HIV, nor could such a patient secrete the virus in the droplets excreted from his or her respiratory tract in coughing or sneezing, or in urine or faeces.

Our scientific knowledge and understanding of how the virus is excreted from an infected person, how it can survive in the interim period, how it can enter the body of a susceptible person and how it establishes infection in that person totally precludes the possibility of these routes, even remotely, being in any way a possibility by which the virus infection can be transmitted.

The risks of HIV transmission in perspective

Educational efforts need to be directed at two goals. On the one hand, high-risk individuals need to be equipped with the means of reducing their risk of acquiring infection through recognized routes of transmission. On the other hand, low-risk individuals need to be reassured about the remoteness of infection via the non-conventional routes. It is true that with HIV, like any other situation in the biological world, it would be impossible to totally rule out very rare, freakish and even bizarre routes of transmission, even though in many of these reported incidents other more conventional routes could not be excluded. It would also be dishonest and counterproductive to categorically deny the occurrence of these freakish incidents of transmission. However, what does need to be put into perspective is that most individuals at work run some small risk of death or injury attached to their work. Life and the pursuit of life's activities does carry its own risk. For example, playing sport, driving of a motor vehicle, flying in an aircraft, or becoming pregnant all carry a measurable risk, all of them far in excess of acquiring HIV infection through these non-conventional routes.

While it would be naive to believe that the fear of so-called 'casual transmission of AIDS' can be totally eliminated, nevertheless those in authority now also need to concentrate educational efforts on how one does *not* get AIDS. If these efforts are at least partially successful, it would contribute greatly to modifying people's attitudes to those infected with the virus. The oft-stated truism which has been applied to many social issues is also very pertinent to AIDS – ignorance breeds fear, fear breeds prejudice and prejudice breeds discrimination, ostracism and eventually hatred.

LIVERPOOL JOHN MOORES UNIVERSITY
LEARNING SERVICES

5

The AIDS test

Laboratory tests are generally performed to confirm clinical diagnoses on patients with symptoms and signs of illness. Occasionally laboratory tests are carried out on asymptomatic persons as part of screening procedures for check-ups or as part of routine examinations, for example for insurance purposes, pre-employment examinations or antenatal screening.

Laboratory tests for HIV infection are similarly carried for routine screening on healthy persons as well as on patients with clinical illness. There is, however, no other diagnostic test which is of such profound significance as the test for HIV infection or, as it is commonly and colloquially known, the 'AIDS test'. The awesome consequences and implications of a positive result make it a unique test amongst all other clinical laboratory tests. Not only is it a confirmation of a terminal illness but it also categorizes the individual as a source of a lethal transmissible virus, who will remain infectious for the rest of his or her life and, in addition, affirms a status that will permanently be a severe social and economic hardship for the rest of that person's life. It is not surprising that issues surrounding this test, such as when it should and should not be done, have been at the centre of some of the most vehement and aggressive debates in the field of medical ethics (which will be discussed more fully in Chapter 8). It is also not unexpected that, once the causal virus had been discovered in 1983 and a method for its propagation described in 1984, a commercially available diagnostic test was developed with unprecedented speed and licensed the following year in 1985. Since then, it has become one of the most sensitive routine tests in all virology. However, given the complexity of the disease, it is not surprising that the reading of laboratory test results may be difficult and tricky and require considerable knowledge and skill for the correct interpretations to be made.

History of the AIDS test

An infectious aetiology of AIDS was suspected soon after the first description of the clinical disease in 1980 and 1981 as discussed in the Introduction. Observations of natural transmission following blood transfusion and also epidemiological studies of sexual transmission soon confirmed that AIDS was due to a transmissible agent. After the earlier contenders – cytomegalovirus, hepatitis B virus and the African swine fever virus – had been eliminated as the cause of AIDS, there began an intense hunt for the responsible agent, driven especially by the critical need for bloodbanks to have a test to screen blood. Following Montagnier's discovery of HIV in 1983 and Gallo's demonstration in 1984 of the propagation of HIV in cell culture, there began one of the most frenetic efforts in medicine to develop a diagnostic test. A number of commercial companies were involved in the race to develop the direly needed, and also promisingly lucrative, test. The first kits for antibody testing became available in April 1985 and later that year commercially produced HIV diagnostic tests were licensed by the FDA of the United States.

These tests were designed on the ELISA (enzyme-linked immunosorbent assay) principle which was, and still is, the most widely used test for detecting viral antibodies in the blood. Initially the antigens used for the tests came from material obtained by chemically digesting the virus particles with enzymes – the so-called viral lysate ELISA tests. These viral lysate tests, also referred to as first generation tests, were of immense benefit in screening blood for HIV infection and dramatically reduced the risk of post-transfusion HIV infection. It was similarly of exceptional value as a clinical diagnostic test for patients with symptoms and for various screening programmes. The early ELISA tests, however, while they were highly sensitive, did suffer from serious drawbacks in terms of specificity, in other words the test frequently registered a positive result in individuals who were not infected. One of the chief reasons for this was the presence of protein materials from the cells on which the virus was grown, contaminating the crude lysate preparations. Many healthy individuals have developed antibodies to these proteins for various reasons, and they would thus erroneously appear positive in the test. In addition, other contaminating materials in the lysates quite often interfered technically with the test, causing it to register a false positive. The presence of false-positive test results was not so noticeable in populations with a high prevalence of true infection, but in those populations where infection was rare it became apparent that the majority of individuals were testing falsely positive and were subsequently shown to be negative. Prospective blood donors were a typical low prevalence population. While sensitivity is clearly a far more critical criterion in terms of safety for a screening procedure in a bloodbank, nevertheless needlessly high false positivity does create serious difficulties because of wastage of blood (which is automatically discarded if it tests positive on screening) as well as the potential for unnecessary loss of blood donors from bloodbank panels and unfortunate and groundless anxiety and anguish to healthy individuals.

It thus soon became clear that people who tested positive on screening tests, and particularly on the early screening tests, ought not to be informed of a positive result until a confirmatory test had also registered positive. A number of laboratory technologies were borrowed from the research laboratories and brought into the clinical diagnostic lay tests. These tests were usually somewhat less sensitive than ELISA but were very much more specific. One of the more commonly used of these confirmatory tests is the Western blot test, which is highly specific as it detects antibodies in the patient's serum that are specifically directed to individual viral proteins. The combination of the highly sensitive ELISA test for screening (carried out in duplicate) followed by the high specificity of the Western blot test became the standard procedure for the diagnosis of infection and is still the norm in a number of countries such as the United States.

However, as valuable as serology was for HIV, the specificity problem of the ELISA test remained a serious problem in the testing of individuals in low-risk groups. A number of technological improvements were made to the first generation tests. Non-specific reactions due to contaminating components from the cell cultures used for propagating the virus were reduced by employing different cell lines for growing the virus. An alternate format for the ELISA test, the so-called competitive ELISA (to be discussed later), also improved the specificity of the test. However, it was the advent of the second generation ELISA tests in the late eighties which has now established the ELISA test as being both highly sensitive as well as highly specific. In these tests, instead of viral lysates being used as the antigenic component, cloned viral proteins produced by recombinant DNA technology, where the specific genes are spliced into producer bacterial or yeast cells, are incorporated into the test. As a result of the use of these exquisitely pure proteins, far fewer false positives occur. More recently, third generation ELISA tests have been developed, further improving on the performance of these diagnostic tests.

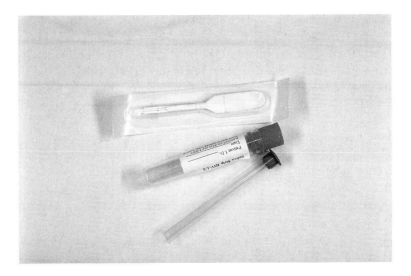

Fig. 5.1 Device for collecting saliva for HIV testing. It consists of an absorbent pad for placing under the tongue to collect a measured amount of saliva, a tube containing a buffered solution to elute out saliva from the pad and an empty tube with a filter on one end to filter out debris from the saliva specimen.

Major technological improvements in the design of ELISA tests have now advanced the performance of this test to a level where sensitivities and specificities of 99.6% and 99.4% respectively are achieved. As a result many countries throughout the world have now adopted the WHO-recommended HIV diagnostic testing strategy, which uses a combination of ELISA tests, rather than relying on expensive secondary tests such as the Western blot for confirmation. The employment of this combination of tests is referred to as the triple ELISA test strategy and it has now become the routine for clinical diagnosis of HIV infection in many countries throughout the world.

Body fluids other than blood, and especially saliva, are being increasingly utilized for initial HIV testing. Devices for collecting saliva commonly consist of an absorbent pad which is placed under the tongue (Fig. 5.1). The appearance of a blue dye in the stem of the device indicates when a sufficient volume of saliva has been collected and the saliva-soaked pad is then sent to a laboratory for testing. The amount of antibody in saliva is very much lower than in serum and modifications to the ELISA test have to be made to detect such low concentrations of antibody. Nevertheless, the sensitivity has been surprisingly good. Positive results do, however, need to be confirmed by conventional ELISA testing on blood before a patient can be diagnosed as being positive. Salivary testing has a number of advantages over blood testing. For example, it is painless, and it can be used where blood is difficult to take, as in the case of children and intravenous drug abusers whose veins are often difficult to access. In addition, saliva specimens avoid the potential hazard of a needle-stick injury to the health care worker.

Cheaper and more rapid tests using techniques other than ELISA have recently come into widespread use. For example, the latex agglutination test, which utilizes antigen stuck onto microscopic latex particles in a suspension. Visible clumps are formed when the particles are agglutinated or stuck together by specific antibodies attaching to the antigens on the beads and linking them together. These tests are considerably cheaper than the ELISA and can give a result within minutes. Although the rapid tests are now being used more and more frequently, especially in hospital wards for quick results, they are relatively limited by their specificity and positive results must be re-tested by ELISA and if necessary a follow-up confirmatory test.

In developing countries various ways to lower the cost of testing have been exploited; for example, in blood donor screening programmes using pools of five to ten blood specimens which are tested as a single specimen, and then re-testing the individual components if the pool is found to be positive.

Principles of laboratory tests for viral diagnosis

There are two fundamental ways in which the laboratory can establish the presence of a viral infection in specimens from a patient – either the virus itself can be detected or the presence of antibodies directed against it or its component proteins can be demonstrated.

Viral detection techniques

Viruses themselves can be detected in specimens by attempting to grow the virus (usually in cell culture), by directly visualizing the virus in a specimen using the electron microscope, or by detecting the presence of the virus' specific antigenic proteins in the specimen.

Many viruses are quite easily and conveniently isolated from a variety of specimens, for example the herpes simplex virus and poliovirus. Virus isolation is commonly performed in routine clinical virology laboratories for these agents. The damage that these viruses cause to cells generally produces a particular and characteristic appearance and their presence can thus quite readily be detected in the cell culture by looking through the microscope. Sometimes further techniques may be needed to demonstrate the presence of virus when they do not produce a characteristic pathological appearance in cell culture – generally the same techniques that are used to detect viral antigen in patients' specimens. However, there are a number of important viruses in humans that either cannot be grown at all in cell culture, for example hepatitis B virus, or only with difficulty in research laboratories but not in the routine clinical diagnostic laboratory, for example rotavirus, the most important single causative agent of infantile gastro-enteritis. These viruses would then need to be detected by alternative means. Viruses that are found in large numbers in body fluids may be visualized directly by the electron microscope; for example, herpes simplex virus in the fluid of fever blisters (cold sores) or genital vesicles, rotavirus in the stools of infants with gastro-enteritis, cytomegalovirus in urine, etc. It has been estimated that at least a million virus particles per millilitre of specimen fluid is necessary for it to be visible in the electron microscope. In addition, while some viruses have very characteristic and easily recognizable shapes under the electron microscope, for example the herpes viruses and rotavirus, many others do not and their diagnosis would need a highly skilled electron microscopist, a specialist not generally available in most clinical virology laboratories.

In the routine clinical virology laboratory the direct detection of many viruses is often carried out by demonstrating the presence of specific viral antigen. This may be done by examining cells secreted by patients into various body fluids, especially respiratory secretions or cells present in the fluid of the blister in herpes simplex or chickenpox. Sometimes these cells assume the characteristic pathological appearance seen in cell culture and merely staining them makes them readily recognizable. Alternatively, the presence of viral antigen inside the cell may be established by adding the appropriate antibody, which would stick specifically to the viral antigen. The antibody which is used is 'labelled' in some way, either by having a fluorescent dye attached to it or else an enzyme that acts on a colourless material to produce a visible coloured dye. If a fluorescent-labelled antibody is used the cells are inspected under a microscope which uses ultraviolet light to make the fluorescent dye glow and become visible. This technique is called immunofluorescence – 'immuno' because it exploits the specificity of the attachment between virus antigen and the particular antibody used as a reagent in the test. The immunofluorescence technique is also commonly used to detect antibodies in serum, by adding the patient's serum to cells infected with the particular virus which are attached to a microscope slide. The technique is very similar if an enzyme producing a coloured dye is latched onto the antibody as a label instead of a fluorescent dye, except that it will then not be necessary to use a special ultraviolet light microscope but an ordinary light microscope to inspect the cells. Examination of cells produced in body secretions for the presence of virus is an important rapid diagnostic test for respiratory infections, especially in children. However, it is only of value when large concentrations of infected cells are shed into body secretions.

The other alternative for demonstrating viral antigen is the use of serological tests (see below) to detect soluble antigen produced in body fluids. The principle of these serological tests is the same as that of tests used for antibody detection except that, in this case, it is the viral antigen in the specimen that is being looked for by using specific antibody which is incorporated into the test. Antigen detection tests are regularly used to screen for the presence of the surface antigen of the hepatitis B virus in blood donors by bloodbanks, as well as in serum from patients with hepatitis. These tests are also commonly used to detect rotavirus antigen in stools of infants with gastro-enteritis, and also in many other applications in routine virology.

More recently, tests to detect nucleic acid are being increasingly utilized for diagnostic purposes, although still not in the routine clinical laboratory. The PCR test has become an extremely important research tool which is now starting to be used in diagnostic laboratories, and has an especially important application for HIV diagnosis. This test has now been developed to be qualitative as well as quantitative. In other words, it is being used to determine whether a particular infectious organism is present or not, as well as to measure the amount of virus in a particular body fluid such as plasma, by quantitating the amount of nucleic acid. It will be discussed in greater detail below.

Viral serology

The term 'serology' is derived from the word 'serum' to denote the process of testing for antibodies in serum (the fluid which remains when blood clots – serum is the same material as plasma except that it lacks the clotting proteins present in plasma which are responsible for the formation of the clot). 'Serology' is now more frequently used in a somewhat broader context to indicate the group of laboratory tests which look either for antibodies (where the test system would incorporate a known specific antigen), or to look for antigen (where the test system would incorporate a known specific antibody) in serum and occasionally other body fluids.

Serological tests are all founded on the principle that a particular antibody will stick to and form a tight bond with the specific antigen that elicited it. This recognition is based on the molecular configuration of the antigen fitting into the complementary configuration on the active binding portion of the antibody, much like a key fits into a lock. Antigens that are subtly different may, on occasion, also react with a particular antibody in much the same way that a set of keys which may be slightly different in their configuration could sometimes still open the same lock. This phenomenon is called cross-reaction. Generally the antigens in the inner portions of the virus tend to cross-react with the inner antigens of viruses within the same group or family. Because there is a finite number of molecular configurations for antigens in nature, as there are a finite number of configurations for keys, occasionally antigens from widely different origins may cross-react, for example a viral antigen and an antigen from a cell protein.

There are a number of designs of serological tests, although all are based on the specificity of the antigen–antibody binding and the tightness of this bond. Thus there are neutralization tests that use live virus to detect specific antibodies in serum. The patient's serum is added to a suspension of virus and if antibodies are present they will bind to the virus and prevent it infecting the cell culture; that is, they will neutralize the virus. To determine the amount of antibody in the serum, a semi-quantitative estimation is made by diluting the patient's serum and repeating the test at each of these various dilutions. The highest dilution that will still neutralize the virus is referred to as the antibody titre and is expressed as the reciprocal of the dilution fraction. This process of dilution is called titration.

The ELISA test, also referred to as the enzyme immunoassay (EIA), is now the most commonly used serological test in virology. The test is based on the stepwise creation of a 'sandwich' of alternate layers of specific antigen and antibody. The format design depends on whether the test is being used to look for antibody or for antigen (Figs. 5.2 and 5.3). In the test for antibody detection the known specific antigen is stuck onto a plastic surface in a specially designed plastic plate or on spherical plastic beads. The patient's serum is then added and if a specific antibody is present it will stick onto the antigen. To now detect the patient's antibody, another antibody called an indicator antibody, which is produced in an animal and directed against the human immunoglobulin molecule (which the antibody comprises), is added. This latter antibody then detects whether the patient's antibody has adhered to the antigen stuck onto the plastic plate or plastic bead. The indicator antibody has an enzyme attached to it (hence the term enzyme immunoassay) which will convert a colourless material added to

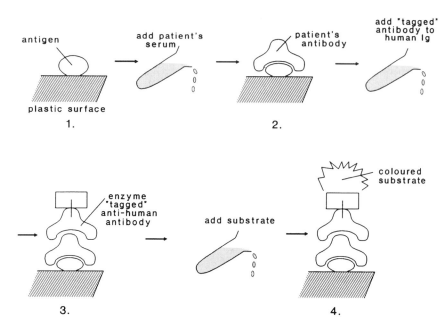

Fig 5.2 Design of ELISA test to detect a specific antibody in patient's serum.

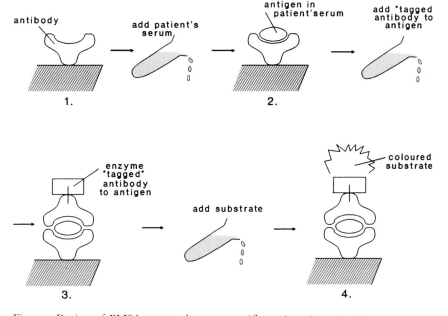

Fig. 5.3 Design of ELISA test to detect a specific antigen in patient's serum.

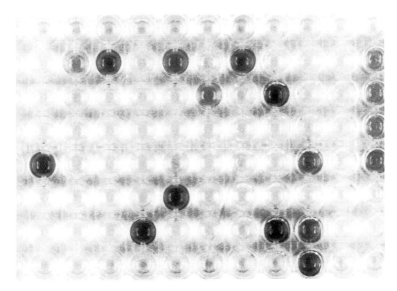

Fig. 5.4 ELISA plate showing positive wells (darkly coloured) with numerous non-coloured negative wells.

the system into a yellow or brown coloured dye. Thus, a positive or negative reaction can be read with the naked eye in the plastic plate or in a test tube housing the plastic bead (Fig. 5.4). The intensity of the colour can also be quantitated in an instrument called a colorimeter and is expressed in terms of optical density (OD). The OD value, which is read on the scale 0–2, is directly proportional to the amount of indicator antibody which is, in turn, directly proportional to the amount of antibody in the patient's serum. The OD reading would thus be equivalent to the titre in the neutralization test.

The test for antigen detection is similar to the antibody test, although the order of the 'sandwich' is reversed. Here, a known specific antibody (usually produced in an animal) directed against the antigen which is being sought is fixed onto a plastic surface and the patient's specimen is then added. If antigen is present it will adhere to the antibody and an indicator antibody with its attached enzyme is then added. The final reaction is similarly read in the colorimeter.

A number of refinements have been brought into the ELISA test to increase the specificity; for example, the competitive ELISA test. In this test a known specific antigen–antibody pair forms part of the components of the test. The patient's serum is then added and the amount of antibody is determined by measuring the degree to which it inhibits the known antigen–antibody reaction by competing with the antibody in the test system for attachment to the antigen in the test. As it is only the active sites that will compete, this test is highly specific.

An important refinement of the ELISA is its use to detect a specific class of antibody. The immunoglobulins, which make up antibodies, are divided into five classes, of which three, IgM (Ig stands for immunoglobulin), IgG and IgA, are the most important for serological tests. The IgM antibodies are produced first in response to infection, after some 10–14 days in the case of acute viral infections, and reach a maximum at about one month. Thereafter there is a gradual decline of IgM antibodies, which eventually disappear after three months. A week or so after the appearance of IgM antibodies, IgG antibodies are found in the blood, reaching a maximum at one to three weeks and then gradually diminishing to a steady low level which remains present for years, sometimes even for a lifetime. Thus, if IgM antibodies are detected, it signifies a current or recent infection (within the past three months), while the presence of IgG signifies that an individual has been infected in the past. In the more chronic and slow-virus infections, IgM and IgG antibodies appear at later time periods and persist for longer periods of time. The IgA antibodies are produced mainly on the mucous membranes of the body and may be detected in these secretions as well as in the bloodstream.

A further important application of the detection of the particular class of specific antibodies in serum is in the diagnosis of infection of infants while in the uterus. The mere detection of antibodies to a particular virus in a young infant does not distinguish between those antibodies which it may have received passively from the mother's bloodstream via the placenta and those which it actively made itself in response to infection. However, it is only the IgG antibodies which cross over through the placenta from the mother to the child. Thus, if IgM or IgA antibodies directed against a particular virus are demonstrated in the infant, it would denote that it was actively infected.

One of the major reasons why the ELISA has become so popular is that it lends itself to automation and bulk-handling of specimens. Thus, in high volume modern laboratories, for example in bloodbank screening, large numbers of specimens can be tested in short periods of time by automated equipment, often using robotics, to dilute serum, add reagents, incubate and read the OD in the colorimeter (Fig. 5.5).

Similar to the ELISA is the radio-immunoassay (RIA), which uses a radioactive isotope as a label instead of an enzyme, and the final result is read in a gamma counter instead of a colorimeter.

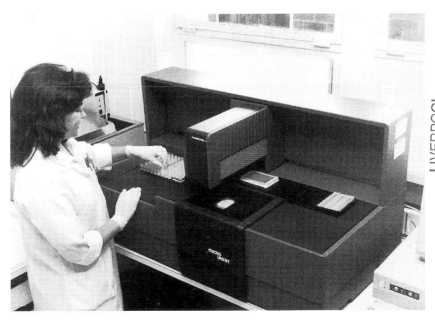

LIVERPOOL
JOHN MOORES UNIVERSITY
AVRIL ROBARTS LRC
TEL. 0151 231 4022

Fig. 5.5 Automated apparatus for diluting and delivering serum and subsequent processing for the ELISA test.

A number of rapid serological tests have been devised which give results in minutes instead of hours or even days, which many of the ELISA tests require. The most widely used of these rapid tests employs microscopic latex beads suspended in a solution which is milky in appearance. A drop of this solution is placed onto a card and a drop of the patient's serum or other type of specimen is then added. The latex particles have antibody fixed onto them if it is antigen which is being looked for, or they would have antigen fixed onto them to detect antibody in the patient's serum. The binding of antigen to antibody links the latex beads to each other to form an extensive lattice network which becomes visible to the naked eye as clumps. A number of latex bead tests have been developed and are becoming increasingly popular because of their convenience, cost, speed and portability.

Recently, more specialized serological tests borrowed from research laboratories have come into use in the clinical laboratory; for example, the Western blot test which is now routinely used in HIV diagnosis. (This will be discussed in greater detail later.)

Reliability and accuracy of serological tests

The performance of a serological test in terms of its accuracy is measured by its sensitivity and specificity. The sensitivity of a test is the measure of its ability to detect specific antibodies when they are truly present; that is, the ability of the test to detect the minutest amount of antibodies in a specimen. The specificity of a test refers to its ability to ignore the presence of antibodies that are not specific; that is, to record a negative result when specific antibodies are absent. In other words, the specificity of a test represents its ability to distinguish specific from non-specific antibodies. Specificity and sensitivity are usually expressed as percentages – the percentage sensitivity of a test being that percentage of infected individuals who are detected by the test, while the percentage specificity of a test is that percentage of non-infected individuals who give a negative test result.

For screening purposes, tests which maximize in sensitivity are generally used, as for example the ELISA test, while, for a definitive diagnosis, tests which may be somewhat less sensitive but are optimally specific are ideally used, as for example the Western blot test.

The laboratory diagnosis of HIV infection

All of the laboratory tests discussed above are used to a lesser or greater extent in the laboratory diagnosis of HIV infection.

Laboratory tests which detect HIV directly

HIV virus can be isolated from the blood (very rarely from other specimens such as genital secretions and extremely rarely from cerebrospinal fluid, tears, saliva and breast milk). A number of techniques for virus isolation have been described, the majority of them based on growing blood cells from a patient together with lymphocytes derived from a healthy donor or from lymphocyte line cells which are propagated indefinitely. The presence of virus in these cultures can be detected, usually after a period of one to two weeks, by the visible appearance (under the light microscope) of syncytia (see Fig. 2.12), or by the detection of soluble p24 antigen (from the core of the virus) in the fluid medium, or by testing for the reverse transcriptase enzyme, or by PCR

In some laboratories success rates of well over 90% are achieved with virus isolation, although in most laboratories that routinely grow virus the isolation rate is somewhat less than that. HIV is far more readily isolated during the acute phase soon after infection, and also after the onset of clinical AIDS disease especially in the terminal stages. The ready isolation of virus in the later stages of infection is a poor prognostic sign, indicating the imminent onset of AIDS, and in patients with AIDS high levels of virus in the blood will signify a deterioration of the patient's condition toward the terminal stages of the illness.

The major reason for isolating virus from patients' specimens is that it provides the laboratory and researchers with an isolate which is then available for further study and characterization, especially subtyping. Virus isolation is essentially of interest to research laboratories and it is really only these laboratories and the large central reference laboratories which are equipped to carry out this test. Virus isolation also requires highly skilled professionals as the technique is difficult and often capricious. It is also expensive, cumbersome and, for security reasons, needs a high level of sophisticated containment facilities to protect workers. In addition to all of this, virus isolation has important shortcomings with regard to its clinical usefulness. Isolation, even in good laboratories, is only successful in somewhat less than 90% of cases and, furthermore, the test itself is time consuming, often taking a number of weeks to get a result. Therefore it is not surprising that virus isolation is seldom carried out in clinical virology laboratories. Other tests to detect the virus have supplanted virus isolation when the indications have arisen to demonstrate the presence of virus in the blood; for example, for prognostic purposes, to monitor therapy and to diagnose intrauterine infection.

(Direct visualization of the virus by electron microscopy is not used as a diagnostic test. Firstly, the virus is rarely found in sufficient quantities in any clinical specimen for it to be visible under the electron microscope, remembering that at least a million particles per millilitre are required for visibility. Secondly, the virus is difficult to recognize in the electron microscope as it does not have a characteristic appearance as do many other viruses, and only few highly skilled and experienced electron microscopists are readily able to recognize HIV.)

At present the most commonly used test in many clinical virology laboratories to directly detect the presence of HIV is the antigen detection test. The ELISA serological technique is used to look for the p24 antigen of the virus in patients' blood. The test is relatively easy to perform, as is the case with conventional ELISA tests used to detect antibodies. However, it does lack sensitivity and if the test is positive it would indicate that substantial amounts of the virus are present in the blood. The antigen detection test has therefore been useful as a prognostic test and also for the monitoring of the patient's response to therapy, especially patients who have

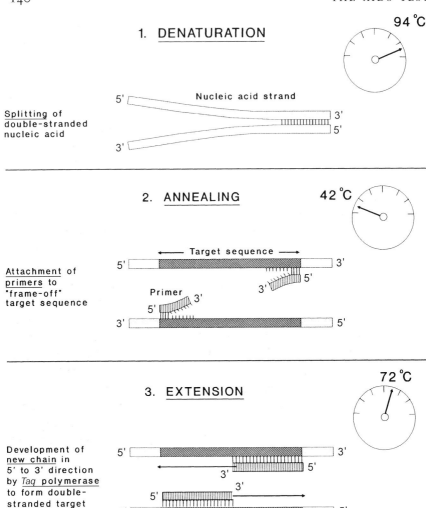

Fig. 5.6 Schematic representation of the polymerase chain reaction (PCR).

high viral loads in their blood and are then found to have cleared the antigen from their blood due to therapy. As a test for infant infection it has
not been particularly useful because of its lack of sensitivity.

The most valuable diagnostic test to directly detect HIV is the PCR which
can be used qualitatively to diagnose the presence of the virus by demonstrating free virus genome, or quantitatively to measure the amount of virus
in a particular body fluid by determining the number of copies of the viral
genome (the viral load test).

The PCR test is able to amplify extremely minute quantities of nucleic acid to reach amounts that can be detectable by probe hybridization. It is therefore incredibly sensitive, being able to detect as little as one target molecule of nucleic acid, or more usually a specific segment thereof, in 10 ml of blood. Expressed another way, the PCR technique is able to detect as little as one fragment of the nucleic acid of HIV in 100 000 host cells. The principle of the test is based on the ability of a particular polymerase enzyme (the enzyme which is responsible for the formation and elongation of nucleic acid) to withstand high temperatures. The PCR procedure consists of three elements (Fig. 5.6). Firstly, the DNA of the host cell is denatured; that is, the two strands are split apart by heating to 90–95°C. This then enables a copy to be made on each of the resultant single strands. In order to do this, the second stage involves cooling the mixture down to 37–50°C and adding a small sequence of nucleic acid corresponding to the specific segment of HIV. This sequence is called a primer as it starts off the elongation process. The primers attach to the corresponding complementary sequences of HIV which have been integrated into the host cell's DNA – a process called annealing. The third stage is for the primer to extend itself to eventually complete the viral nucleic acid segment that is being looked for. This primer extension is carried out by the unique thermostable polymerase enzyme at a high temperature of 67–72°C. When the extension is complete, the mixture is again heated up to 90–95°C and the whole cycle is then repeated. Thus, multiple cycles of denaturation, annealing and polymerization would take place by merely switching temperatures from 94°C to 42°C to 72°C. With each cycle the number of copies of the target sequence increases exponentially so that, in theory, after 20–30 cycles a billion copies could be made in less than three hours. Thus, more than ample amounts of amplified specific DNA can be made from very tiny amounts of starting material.

The exquisite sensitivity of the PCR, while it has clearly been of outstanding benefit in the diagnosis of HIV especially as the virus is usually in such minute amounts in clinical specimens, has intrinsic difficulties, principally with regard to specificity. The primer pairs (one for each strand of DNA) have to be very carefully chosen as any overlapping and hybridization with a non-viral portion of nucleic acid would be greatly amplified and easily give a false-positive result. So sensitive is the test that even the minutest amounts of nucleic acid, which could be carried in the air or contaminate equipment or hands, can cause false positives and usually the amplification steps are carried out in a room dedicated for this purpose. As a result of the problems of non-specificity of the test, the PCR should still be carried out only in those laboratories that have the appropriate experience and skills to carry out and interpret the test appropriately. The PCR test can be used to detect HIV RNA which reflects free virus in a particular body fluid, and also HIV DNA in cells, especially lymphocytes, denoting virus that is integrated into the cell's chromosome.

One of the most important developments in the management of HIV infection in recent times has been the advent of the diagnostic tests which measure the amount of virus in body fluids, especially plasma. These tests have become known as the viral load tests. They have contributed greatly to the understanding of the mechanisms of HIV disease. In particular they have revealed that during the so-called 'clinically silent' phase of the disease the virus is, in fact, actively and vigorously replicating in various sites of the body, in particular the lymphoid organs. Here some ten billion or so virus particles are being produced daily. This has strongly supported the initiation of early antiviral therapy to reduce the viral load before it builds up to high levels with resultant extensive destruction of CD4 lymphocytes.

The viral load test measures the amount of HIV RNA in plasma and is also, on occasion, used to quantitate virus in other body fluids for diagnostic or research purposes. At present there are three clinical diagnostic tests for measuring HIV RNA. Firstly, there is the PCR-based amplification test. In this technique virus RNA is reverse transcribed into DNA which is amplified together with a control specimen consisting of a known number of copies of DNA. Hence, by comparing the signal reading of the test with that of the control specimen, the number of copies of HIV RNA in the patient's specimen can be calculated with a fair degree of precision. The second technique is called the branched DNA (bDNA) because, in this test, it is the signal which is amplified rather than the HIV RNA. This is done by producing an extensive branched chain lattice consisting of nucleotide molecules. The intensity of signal from the probe is directly proportional to the amount of HIV RNA in the sample. The third technique, used somewhat less frequently than the other two, is called nucleic acid sequence-based amplification (NASBA).

The viral load tests have become the most important diagnostic tests for assessing the prognosis of a patient as well as for monitoring response to therapy. These tests are able to provide precise and accurate measurements of the number of copies of the virus (that is, the number of virus particles) per millilitre of plasma. For prognostic purposes, the baseline determination of the number of virus copies in the plasma has proven to be a reliable predictor of the outcome of the disease course in that patient. Furthermore, evidence of progression of disease can be monitored by repeating the viral load test at six-monthly intervals. Viral load tests are also of great value in assessing the response to antiviral therapy. Here also, six-monthly viral load determinations are able to provide important guidelines to the doctor as to whether the drug regimen should be changed or maintained. The test can also provide an early warning indication of drug failure.

HIV serology

The spectrum of serological tests used in virology in general have also been utilized for HIV serology. However, it is the ELISA test which still remains by far the most widely used of all the clinical laboratory tests for HIV infection.

As mentioned above, the ELISA test has undergone a number of improvements from the first generation viral lysate tests to the second generation recombinant antigen tests. A number of formats have been designed by different commercial kit manufacturers. Some ELISA tests incorporate more layers into the 'sandwich', others utilize the competitive principle. The choice of kit used by a clinical virology laboratory is often based on the experience of that laboratory, the type of automated equipment that is available and the compatibility with other diagnostic tests in the laboratory. Most laboratories would use more than one type of kit at any particular time.

More recently a variety of rapid diagnostic tests have been developed and marketed, and are being extensively used not only in virology laboratories but also by practising physicians, in hospitals and side-wards, and even as home testing kits to be used by lay persons. (Regulations in the United Kingdom have made it an offence to sell these kits to the public or to provide HIV testing services other than through a registered medical practitioner. In the USA, however, the FDA has permitted, amid some considerable controversy, the sale of home-testing kits to the lay public.) Rapid tests which produce a result within minutes are either based on the particle agglutination principle, which uses microscopic latex beads or similar particles, or on the immunoblot principle. In the latter, HIV antigen is blotted onto an absorbent paper such as nitrocellulose paper, and a drop of specimen is then placed onto the blot. Attachment of antibodies to antigen is demonstrated by a colour reaction which develops when a labelled indicator antibody is added. All of these rapid tests have very major advantages in terms of speed, cost, convenience and portability. However, they are of lower specificity than the ELISA test and, especially in unskilled hands, may yield a prohibitively high rate of false positivity.

A number of confirmatory tests for HIV infection have been developed and are used in various clinical virology laboratories. In the USA, the most commonly used confirmatory test is the Western blot. The name 'Western blot' has a rather quaint origin. The original blot test, called the Southern blot, was described by Dr Edward Southern and was used to detect DNA by blotting material onto nitrocellulose paper and probing this blot for specific sequences of DNA. A similar blot was then developed for the detection of RNA and was named, in an attempt to inject some humour into the dullness of biochemistry, the Northern blot. So it was, that when a similar blot was designed for detecting proteins it was not too unpredictably called the Western blot!

The purpose of the HIV Western blot test is to detect antibodies in the patient's serum which react with the specific proteins of HIV. The pattern which is produced by the reaction of antibodies in the patient's serum to the various proteins of the virus provides a very specific picture which is indicative of infection with the virus. The test itself consists of two parts: firstly, the digestive splitting of the virus into its constituent proteins, separating them out and blotting them onto nitrocellulose paper, and, secondly, using these proteins to test for the presence of specific antibodies directed against them.

To split and separate the proteins of the virus, the virus particles are first digested with an enzyme which breaks up the capsid or protein shell of the virus, and produces a solution of the discrete viral proteins. These proteins are then put into a jelly-like material called polyacrylamide gel on a glass plate, and an electric current is passed through which separates out the individual proteins according to their molecular weight and electric charge (a process called electrophoresis) (Fig. 5.7). A sheet of nitrocellulose paper is then placed onto the gel and the protein bands are then blotted onto the paper. The paper with its lines of protein blots is then cut into thin strips, each strip containing all the separated protein bands. These strips function as the starting reagent for the detection of antibodies to individual viral proteins in the patient's serum. In practice, commercial Western blot kits consist of these nitrocellulose strips with pre-blotted protein bands.

The second stage of the Western blot is essentially the same as a sandwich ELISA test. The first layer (corresponding to the fixed antigen in the ELISA test to detect antibodies) is the virus protein antigen band on the nitrocellulose paper. The patient's serum is then placed onto the paper and an enzyme-labelled indicator antibody is added on top of that. The final stage is the addition of the colourless substrate which is converted to a

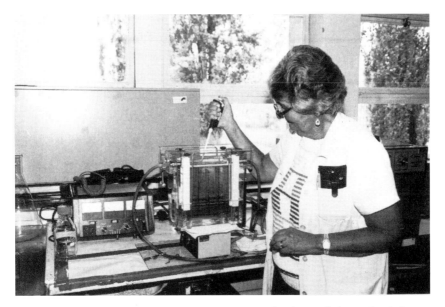

Fig. 5.7 Virus material that has been enzymatically digested, being loaded onto a gel apparatus to be electrically separated (electrophoresis) into its constituent proteins in the Western blot test.

coloured material by the enzyme (provided that the indicator antibody has attached to the patient's antibody which, in turn, has recognized and attached to the particular band on the nitrocellulose strip). The presence of the specific antibody is thus indicated by a dark coloured band (blue or brown) corresponding to the position of the indicator antibody attached to the nitrocellulose strip (Fig. 5.8).

Unfortunately, up to the present time, no international consensus has been reached as to what combination of bands would define a positive result. Various bodies, such as the Centers for Disease Control, WHO, the American Red Cross and others, have each devised their own diagnostic definitions for positivity. The three groups of proteins which are detected by Western blot are those of the envelope (*env*), the core or group specific antigen (*gag*) and the polymerase enzyme (*pol*) (Fig. 5.9). The three envelope glycoproteins are gp160, the large precursor molecule which is then split into the two component *env* proteins – the outermost spike, gp120, and the transmembrane protein, gp41. The *env* proteins are the most specific of the viral proteins and, by all of the Western blot diagnostic definitions, have to be present for a diagnosis to be made. In some definitions, even if the envelope proteins are the only bands present, the minimal presence

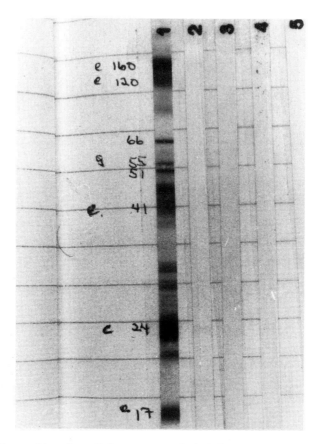

Fig. 5.8 Western blot nitrocellulose strips with dark bands indicating the presence of antibodies in patient's serum directed against the corresponding individual viral proteins.

of both *env* proteins would constitute a positive diagnosis. The main *gag* protein is the precursor protein, p55, which is split into its constituent p18 and p24 proteins. The *gag* proteins are not as specific as the *env* proteins, and some cross-reactivity occurs with other retroviruses. They are generally the first antibodies to appear in a patient with HIV infection and also the first to disappear in advanced cases of AIDS. Some Western blot diagnostic definitions require at least one *gag* protein for a positive diagnosis to be made. The *pol* proteins, p31, p51 and p66 are the least important proteins for diagnosis. They also cross-react with other retroviruses and only one Western blot diagnostic definition insists on a member of this group being present for a positive diagnosis.

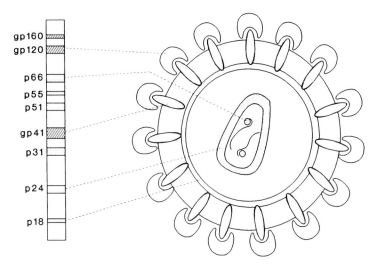

gp160
gp120
p66
p55
p51
gp41
p31
p24
p18

Fig. 5.9 Schematic view of HIV-1 virus (right) with the corresponding proteins demonstrable on a nitrocellulose Western blot strip (left).

The absence of any band on the Western blot means that the patient lacks all antibodies and is serologically negative for HIV infection. The presence of bands which satisfy the definition used by a particular laboratory would indicate a confirmed positive result. However, about 20–40% of sera sent for confirmation to laboratories in developed countries, and probably an even higher percentage in Africa, produce some bands on Western blot but an insufficient number to meet the diagnostic definition for positivity. Such a result is called an indeterminate result and this has been a major source of confusion and concern with regard to its interpretation and meaning. The majority of indeterminate results occurring in high-risk individuals are indicative of early infection. For example, as p24 antibodies are the earliest of the specific antibodies to appear, an isolated p24 band without *env* protein bands would be interpreted as an indeterminate result. In low-risk individuals the origin of these isolated protein bands is not known and their significance is uncertain. In African sera, excessive globulins are frequently present, causing a phenomenon called 'sticky sera', as these proteins appear to adhere non-specifically in serological tests producing false-positive results. In the Western blot test, 'sticky sera' are a frequent cause of indeterminate results. Occasionally an indeterminate Western blot result is due to infection with a cross-reacting retrovirus such as HIV-2 or HTLV-I.

Individuals whose blood gives an indeterminate Western blot result are cautioned not to donate blood and are counselled with regard to the use of condoms in their sexual relationships. Their sera are re-tested after six months and if they have reverted to negativity they are reassured. If the serum still gives an indeterminate Western blot result and they are low-risk individuals, they are also generally reassured and the indeterminate results are regarded as a harmless anomaly. The majority of these indeter-minate Western blot patterns eventually disappear. High-risk individuals would, however, be re-tested at six months and, if negative, they would continue to be monitored for infection.

The problem of the indeterminate result, however, still remains and causes a great deal of uncertainty and anguish. It has also been a major reason, together with the cost factor, for the calls by a number of author-ities for the removal of the Western blot as a diagnostic test and its replace-ment by the use of multiple ELISA tests. Many countries in the world have now adopted a strategy of using ELISA tests alone for diagnostic testing in place of the combination of an ELISA test for initial testing followed by Western blot for confirmation.

The laboratory diagnosis of HIV-2

As HIV-2 is still rare outside West Africa, Angola and Mozambique, relatively little attention has been given to its diagnosis in most other countries. Because of cross-reactions between the core proteins of the two viruses, ELISA tests for HIV-1 will diagnose an HIV-2 infection in 30–80% of cases. There are, however, specific commercial ELISA kits for HIV-2, and frequently a combination kit of HIV-1 and HIV-2 is used for screen-ing purposes. Combined HIV-1/HIV-2 kits have now been recommended for the routine screening in bloodbanks in the USA. There are also specific Western blot kits for further confirmation.

Tests for the evaluation of immunological function

In addition to tests to establish a diagnosis of HIV infection, the measure-ment of the degree of suppression of immune function forms a major part of the laboratory evaluation of an HIV-infected individual, and is also essential in assessing the response of the patient to therapy. There are two types of laboratory tests of immune function, those which enumerate the spe-cific subsets of lymphocytes and those which assess the functional capacity of the lymphocyte.

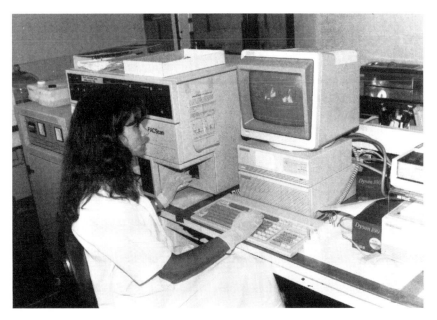

Fi. 5.10 Flow cytometer used to enumerate lymphocyte subsets identified by antibodies to specific cell surface markers. (See also Fig. 3.3.)

Lymphocyte enumeration (subset enumeration)

The most important parameter of immune function to be evaluated is the enumeration of the patient's lymphocytes, as the hallmark of HIV infection is the profound depletion of CD4 lymphocytes. A crude initial estimation of this depletion may be obtained from the count of the total lymphocyte population. However, to obtain a more precise measure of HIV immuno-suppression, an enumeration of the subsets of lymphocytes, specifically the CD4 lymphocytes, must be carried out. This is usually done by 'tagging' these lymphocytes with a fluorescent-labelled antibody directed against the CD4 and CD8 antigens as well as other surface antigens (see Fig. 3.3). The number of lymphocytes that are 'tagged' can then be enumerated in an automated counting apparatus called a flow cytometer (Fig. 5.10).

The normal count of CD4 lymphocytes is about 1000 cells per cubic millimeter. In HIV infection the count drops markedly and usually by the time it reaches less than 200 cells per cubic millimetre, AIDS disease is present or imminent. In the newest of the clinical classifications of AIDS suggested by the CDC, the proposal is made that the finding of a CD4 lymphocyte count of less than 200 cells per cubic millimetre should be a criterion for the diagnosis of AIDS. The cut-off value of less than 200 cells per cubic millimetre has also been used as a criterion for zidovudine treatment in asymptomatically infected persons.

In addition to the enumeration of CD4 lymphocytes, the CD8 or suppressor lymphocyte is also frequently enumerated in a flow cytometer and the ratio of CD4 to CD8 lymphocytes is also an important diagnostic test. In healthy persons there are some four times as many CD4 lymphocytes as CD8 lymphocytes. With the depletion of the CD4 lymphocyte this ratio drops and eventually reverses, as the number of CD8 lymphocytes overtakes that of CD4 lymphocytes. The reversal of the CD4:CD8 lymphocyte ratio is of similar significance to the drop in the absolute CD4 count to below 200 cells per cubic millimetre. In practice the CD4:CD8 ratio has been of much lesser value, in terms of prognosis, than the absolute CD4 lymphocyte count.

Functional analysis of lymphocytes

A number of tests of lymphocyte function are routinely carried out in immunology laboratories. These include the T-lymphocyte cytotoxicity test, that is the test to determine the functional ability of lymphocytes to kill cells. The lymphocyte blast transformation test measures the ability of lymphocytes to change their morphology in response to immune stimulation. Skin testing measures the cellular immune response by the production of a delayed hypersensitivity reaction to various challenge antigens injected into the skin, which the individual may have been exposed to. These lymphocyte functional tests are time consuming and expensive and do not offer any more useful information than lymphocyte enumeration. Skin tests are less reliable as an indicator of immunosuppression than is lymphocyte enumeration.

Surrogate markers

A number of biochemical tests indicative of immune activation are commonly used in the monitoring of AIDS patients. The two most widely used of these are the β-2 (beta-2) microglobulin and neopterin.

β-2 Microglobulin is part of an antigen found on the surface of cells. Levels of this protein are elevated in the blood in association with activation of lymphocytes, and correlate strongly with the more rapid deterioration towards the onset of AIDS. Neopterin, a chemical derivative of the nucleic acid building blocks, is produced mainly by monocytes and macrophages. Raised levels of this material, measured in serum or urine, similarly indicate a worsening of the prognosis and a deterioration towards AIDS.

With the increasingly widespread use of viral load measurement to assess prognosis and response to therapy, these biochemical tests are being less frequently utilized.

Laboratory tests in practice

Diagnostic testing

Laboratory tests for HIV are performed on healthy asymptomatic individuals as well as on clinically ill patients where HIV-related disease may be suspected. Healthy persons request HIV testing generally because they are concerned about being infected for a variety of reasons ranging from past sexual misdemeanours to exaggerated anxieties of having contracted the infection. These individuals are often referred to as the 'worried well' and the HIV test serves the valuable purpose of obtaining the reassurance of a negative result. Similarly, many HIV tests are carried out on individuals who have had definite exposures such as sexual contact with a high-risk person, or a needle-stick exposure by a health care worker. The average time from exposure to the development of antibodies is conventionally given as six to eight weeks, although shorter periods are common when individuals have been followed up after an exposure. The protocol which is generally followed for the serological checking of persons after possible exposure to HIV involves an early specimen taken as soon as possible to ensure that the individual is not already infected, and then a specimen at about two months after exposure. If both are negative a further specimen could be taken at six months to exclude late seroconversion (development of antibodies). A negative result at six months after exposure should provide reasonable reassurance, as delayed seroconversions after this time, although they have been reported, are very rare.

Serological testing for HIV is now also one of the most frequently performed laboratory examinations in clinically ill patients. Infection with HIV can manifest with a variety of signs and symptoms and the clinical indications to perform an HIV test are very wide. These would include patients manifesting with an acute influenza-like illness with lymph gland swelling, patients with prolonged unexplained weight loss or chronic fever or diarrhoea, patients with the unusual infections associated with AIDS and unexplained behavioural changes. Clearly the suspicion of HIV as the cause for a clinical presentation is very much strengthened if the patient practises high-risk activities.

The initial routine HIV test is an ELISA test. If this is negative the individual may be reassured and generally no further testing is needed because of its very high sensitivity. A positive ELISA is usually referred to as being 'reactive' rather than 'positive', as no definitive positive diagnosis can be made on a single ELISA test. Following a reactive result, the test is then repeated using an ELISA from a different manufacturer. If it is repeatedly reactive, the specimen is tested a third time by ELISA – the triple ELISA strategy. Alternatively, in some countries such as the USA it is then forwarded for a confirmatory test, usually the Western blot. A positive result in all three ELISA tests or a positive Western blot would be regarded as being diagnostic of HIV infection. However, because of the risk of clerical errors in any large laboratory, it is usual to request another fresh specimen from the patient, and only if this second specimen is also confirmed to be positive would the patient be diagnosed as being infected.

Screening programmes

Screening for HIV infection is carried out for various purposes. Many employer organizations routinely screen prospective employees, although considerable ethical difficulties arise from this practice (to be considered later in Chapter 8). The insurance and related industries require routine HIV screening of applicants for policies above a certain value. In many parts of the world antenatal screening is an important component of the routine care of pregnant women.

Screening programmes frequently involve high-volume automated ELISA testing of large numbers of specimens. The finding of a reactive specimen from a screening programme should be viewed only as an indication for such a person to report for a more formal HIV test on a separate specimen of blood.

Bloodbank screening

As already mentioned, the screening of donated blood has dramatically reduced the incidence of new HIV infections from transfusion to a point where it is now very rare for infection to occur from screened blood. Highly automated ELISA testing equipment is used by most bloodbanks where large numbers of specimens are screened. Donors whose blood is reactive on screening should be referred to a clinic for formal testing as outlined above in 'Diagnostic testing'.

In developing countries, the cost of screening blood with commercial ELISA kits is often prohibitively high, and in much of the poorer sections of the world little or no screening can be carried out. Costs may, however, be significantly reduced if the blood specimens are pooled into groups of five, and each pool tested as if it were a single specimen. If a pool is found to be reactive, then the individual specimens comprising it can be separately tested. However, as valuable as pooling is for cutting costs, it is really only economically advantageous if the prevalence of HIV in the potential donor population is less than 2%, otherwise too many of the pools turn out to be reactive for it to be cost-saving. Unfortunately, in many developing countries of the world with high HIV prevalences, pooling often would not alleviate the high cost of routine blood screening.

A continuing source of anxiety for bloodbanks is the possibility that infected individuals who are antibody negative could donate blood. Absence of antibodies occurs at two stages of HIV infection – the terminal stages, when it would be highly unlikely that such an individual would donate blood and, more importantly, during the 'window period' stage before antibodies have developed, which generally lasts up to four to eight weeks after infection. Unfortunately, there have been no practical diagnostic solutions to the problem of the 'window period'. Theoretically, the antigen detection ELISA test should have a role in this kind of screening, but it is unfortunately far too insensitive and is, in fact, not often positive in the 'window period'. Virus cultures would, of course, be totally impractical as a screening test for any sizeable number of specimens. The PCR technique is being investigated as a diagnostic possibility but it is still far too expensive and cumbersome for large-scale screening, even if specimens were to be pooled. PCR, if it does become practical, could reduce the 'window period' down to two weeks. However, as mentioned in Chapter 4, the risk of infection from blood donated during the 'window period' of time is of the order of one in a million in developed countries, although in many developing countries in Africa and Asia the risk may be as high as 1 in 10 000 or less.

Testing for surveillance purposes

Prevalence studies are an intrinsic component of the national and international monitoring of the HIV epidemic. Specimens are generally sampled from representative sections of the population, which would convey useful information regarding the epidemiology of HIV. Thus, sentinel groups such as high-risk attenders of sexually transmitted diseases clinics or mothers attending antenatal clinics, or low-risk prospective blood donors could all provide very useful information regarding the prevalence of HIV in different sections of the population and thus contribute to an overall picture of the epidemic in that region. Information generated from the screening of prospective blood donors is automatically available and merely needs to be obtained from the bloodbanks and then analysed. Sampling of other groups requires active planning in terms of having an adequate size of sample which is randomly selected and sufficiently representative. This kind of surveillance is often referred to as active surveillance in contrast to the passive surveillance of blood donors where the data have already been generated and merely need to be collected and analysed. In active surveillance studies the specimens that are obtained are usually unlinked and anonymous, in other words they carry no labels and there is no way in which a person can be linked to a specimen or can be identified. These studies have therefore no role in the diagnosis of infection in individuals, and the ethical stringencies that apply to patient testing are therefore considerably more relaxed. It would, thus, not be necessary to do confirmatory tests on reactive specimens as the error rate with the ELISA test is small enough not to materially affect the validity of the prevalence figures. It would also, in cases where the prevalence of infection is low, be satisfactory and cost-effective to pool specimens, especially if large numbers are being examined, to cut costs.

HIV diagnosis in infants

Infants born to HIV-infected mothers have, on average, a 30% chance of being actively infected while in the uterus or during birth. Diagnosis of infection in the infant is, however, complicated by the fact that the antibodies in the mother's bloodstream cross the placenta into the infant's bloodstream. Therefore, serological detection of antibodies in the infant does not distinguish between those antibodies which the infant would have made in response to infection and those which it acquired passively from its mother. Maternal antibodies may remain and be detectable in the infant's bloodstream for up to 15 months after birth and thus conventional serological tests would be unable to diagnose infection in infancy.

As it is only the IgG class of antibodies that is able to cross from the mother to the infant, earlier attempts were made to modify HIV serological tests such as the ELISA to detect specific IgM antibodies which, if they are present, would indicate that the infant had been infected as they could not have come from the mother. (The detection of specific IgM antibodies is commonly used to diagnose congenital infections by a number of viruses, such as rubella and cytomegalovirus.) Unfortunately, IgM-specific tests have not been successful for diagnosing HIV infection. There was, for a time, some interest in the development of a specific HIV IgA test, especially the adaptation of the Western blot to detect IgA antibodies.

At present the diagnosis of the infant has mainly involved viral detection tests rather than serology. Antigen detection was found to be too insensitive and virus culture was both insensitive as well as expensive and time consuming. Diagnosis of infant infection is generally done by PCR and this is one of the most important applications of the PCR test. Minute amounts of HIV nucleic acid may be detected in the infant's blood by the PCR technique and quantitative PCR is used to measure the viral load in the infant's blood to assess prognosis.

Patient monitoring

As discussed previously, quantitation of HIV RNA in the patient's plasma (the viral load test) has become a crucial diagnostic test in the management of HIV disease. It is the most accurate test for determining the prognosis of the patient as well as for monitoring the patient's response to therapy. For prognostication it provides a good indication of the risk of disease progression. It has been shown that after the acute infection the mass of HIV RNA settles down to a level often referred to as the 'set point'. If a test is carried out at this early stage of infection it could give a good idea of the expected duration of the asymptomatic period as well as the expected survival time of that individual. If the test is done at a later stage it provides a reliable indication of the risk of progression of the disease. With respect to monitoring of antiviral therapy, the viral load test provides the doctor with important guidelines as to the efficacy of therapy as well as sounding an early warning if the therapy is failing. In general, a viral load test should be done when the patient is first seen to provide a baseline value. The patient should then be monitored at intervals of three to six months (although shorter intervals would be needed if the clinical condition deteriorates or if therapy is changed).

The CD4 lymphocyte count and the enumeration of lymphocyte subsets are complementary tests to the viral load test and would generally be done together with it. Their role in patient management is somewhat different to that of the viral load test. The CD4 lymphocyte count is a measure of the immunological status of the patient and therefore determines the stage of disease that the patient has reached. (The main pathological effect of HIV disease is the depletion of CD4 lymphocytes.) For example, the CD4 counts are used as indicators for when to commence prophylaxis against opportunistic infections. A graphic analogy of the relative contributions of these two important tests is that of a speeding train rushing towards a precipice. The viral load test would represent the speed of the train while the CD4 lymphocyte count would be the milestone markers measuring out the distance before the train reaches the precipice.

Benefits of the 'AIDS test'

The 'AIDS test' has virtually since its inception and widespread use drawn considerable controversy and firm opposition from many quarters. There is considerable fear that a positive diagnosis would itself create symptoms because of the intense emotional anxiety associated with HIV infection. There is also a fear that the confidentiality of the test results could be lost with the frightful social and economic consequences which may occur. Many activist groups have vigorously campaigned against people going for HIV testing because of the fear of discrimination and victimization. It is like no other test in clinical medicine, so it is imperative that adequate psychological preparation is provided before the test is carried out. Should the test prove to be positive, the result must be conveyed to the patient by a skilled counsellor. All too often HIV tests are carried out without sufficient pre-test counselling and, even worse, positive results are often provided cursorily and unsympathetically to patients.

However, if adequate pre- and post-test counselling is provided and also if confidentiality is assured, there are many benefits to the individual in having the AIDS test. Firstly, the obvious optimistic benefit is that of a negative result providing dramatic relief from anxiety and giving desperately needed reassurance. Secondly, even a positive result will be of psychological help by removing the anxiety of uncertainty. Thirdly, the individual who knows he or she is positive can plan a lifestyle that could delay the onset of AIDS. There is considerable evidence that asymptomatically infected individuals who pursue a healthy lifestyle with good dietary habits and sufficient exercise, and a motivated psychological outlook, can postpone the onset of AIDS. Fourthly, the awareness of being HIV positive would give the individual the benefit of a heightened awareness in recognizing signs of opportunistic infections at an early stage, when treatment is more likely to be effective. Fifthly, with the progress being made in early specific antiviral treatment (see Chapter 6), having a knowledge of being HIV positive would enable an individual to benefit from the possible advantages of antiviral treatment at a stage of the infection where very significant benefits could be achieved. Sixthly, the knowledge of HIV positivity would clearly have a major role to play in the prevention of HIV transmission by, for example, alerting infected individuals to avoid donating blood, to practise safe sex or avoid pregnancy. Finally, the knowledge of being HIV positive is something which many infected individuals would not want withheld from them. Knowing they are positive would enable them to make appropriate long-term plans for their own futures and those of their dependants.

6

The anti-AIDS drugs

A general sense of frustration is often felt at the apparent slowness in developing drugs to cure viral infections. That the human race, which was able to put a man on the moon, is seemingly unable to develop a cure for the common cold appears to be quite unacceptable. The discovery of the HIV virus in 1983 and 1984 brought with it a sense of euphoria that, having identified the enemy, it would now be but a matter of time before such a puny adversary was wiped out by the might of human technological armaments. However, the number of effective drugs able to treat viral infections is still small and comparatively few viruses (mainly some members of the herpes virus family and now, to an increasing extent, HIV) are amenable to antiviral therapy. This is in marked contrast to the wide spectrum of highly effective antibiotics and antimicrobial drugs which are available for the treatment of all bacterial infections. Why antiviral drug development is still only at such a rudimentary stage as compared to antibiotic therapy needs now to be examined, in order to appreciate the enormous difficulties involved in the development of effective agents to treat HIV infection.

The development of antiviral drugs

The theoretical basis of antimicrobial drugs

Microbes, be they viruses, bacteria, fungi or parasites, all share common designs of chemical and physical structures consistent with all life forms. There are many chemical substances that can kill or inactivate all microbes and a number of such materials are effective in disinfecting inanimate objects such as, for example, the surface of tables and floors in operating theatres, and surgical instruments. Many of these materials can also be used for disinfecting the outer surfaces of the body; for example, alcohol solutions, iodine-containing solutions, detergents and other chemicals, which are commonly employed to disinfect wounds, sterilize skin before an operation, disinfect a surgeon's hands, in mouthwashes, douches, eye preparations and so on. Provided they remain on the surface of the body and do not come into contact with the cells inside the body, and also provided they are not locally irritating, they do no harm and are active in destroying microbes. This they do by a direct toxic effect on the proteins of microbial cells or viruses, or on their nucleic acids, or membranes. However, their activities are non-specific and non-selective and they can damage and destroy the proteins, nucleic acids and membranes of any living organism including the cells of the host body. Thus, they could not be used to treat infections inside the body where they might come into contact with living cells which could likewise be damaged or destroyed. For a drug to be utilizable for the treatment of infections in the body, it needs to be active against the microbe but not the cells of the host body. This selective activity forms the basis of antimicrobial drug design, and it is also the important difference between an antiseptic or disinfectant, which can only be used on the surface of the body, and an antimicrobial drug, which can also be taken internally. Furthermore, the value of an antimicrobial drug will be proportional to its selectivity in terms of its effectiveness against the microbe on the one hand and its lack of toxicity against the host body's cells on the other. Occasionally this gap of selectivity may not be wide enough and such a drug may be quite toxic to both virus and host. Nevertheless it may still be quite useful therapeutically, provided that its use is confined to the surface of the body. Thus, antimicrobial drugs may be employed for use on the surfaces of the body, referred to as topical or localized use, or they may be administered by injection or orally, to be distributed throughout the body, called systemic use. There is no drug which is completely safe and all have had some side-effects reported. Essentially, the decision to use any drug is taken on balance of the benefits of the drug outweighing its potential side-effects. In the designing of new drugs, it is this balance of effectiveness versus potential toxicity which governs the feasibility and value of a future drug.

The development of antibacterial agents

One of the major reasons why antibacterial agents are so plentiful, so effective and usually so safe is that bacteria are so different structurally and biochemically to mammalian or human cells. The majority of bacteria are able to survive and multiply outside living cells and also have a sturdy cell wall. This cell wall is not present in mammalian cells, and therefore offers itself as a selective target to antibiotics such as penicillin and others related to it. (Side-effects due to the penicillins are due to other properties of the drug, not related directly to its mode of action.) Similarly, the structure and functioning of bacterial ribosomes (the organelles inside the cells responsible for the manufacture of proteins) are markedly different from those of the host cell's ribosomes and, again, offer themselves as targets for the selective activity of antibiotics such as the tetracyclines. There are many other examples where the metabolic pathways or the structural components of bacteria are so different from those of the host cells that they can be exploited in devising drugs that can act selectively on bacteria with little or no effect on the functioning of the cell. In many cases antibacterial drugs are so effective that they eliminate the invading organisms completely. These drugs are referred to as bacteriocidal agents. In some situations the drug merely reduces the load of the organisms by preventing any further multiplication, and the body's immune response is then responsible for the elimination of the rest of the organisms. These agents are referred to as bacteriostatic agents.

The difficulties in the development of antiviral agents

In contrast to antibacterial drugs, the development of antiviral agents faces far greater obstacles. In fact, up until a few decades ago, it was widely thought that it would not be possible to develop antiviral drugs to any significant extent because of the overlap between the biochemical processes of viruses and those of cells, and it would thus be virtually impossible to design chemical agents that would be sufficiently selective to be therapeutically useful.

There are some viruses, such as herpes, that do have biochemical pathways which are unique to these viruses and are not found in the host cell. These pathways have offered the drug designer an opportunity to target drugs to act specifically on the viruses without inflicting damage to the cell as seen, for example, in the antiviral drug acyclovir (Zovirax®). This substance is inactive as it is and only becomes activated when a chemical group, called a phosphate, is coupled to it by an enzyme called kinase. This initial activation step can virtually exclusively only be carried out by the kinase from herpes virus, and hardly at all by the kinases of the cell. As a result this drug is very active against the virus and has little toxicity for the host. Unfortunately, there are few other examples of antiviral agents with such remarkable selectivity and there are also relatively few other viruses which have, to date, offered such targets for the drug designer's ingenuity. The repertoire of viruses that are being targeted for development of new antiviral drugs has recently expanded somewhat and now includes viruses such as those that cause hepatitis and influenza. The spectrum of usable drugs, however, still remains relatively limited.

A further difficulty with antiviral therapy is the fact that with acute virus infections, the clinical presentation of disease, that is when the patient is conscious of being infected with the virus, only occurs at a relatively late stage during the course of infection, often when virus replication has almost ceased. Any potential benefit of antiviral therapy would then have already passed. As a corollary to this, antiviral therapy, to be effective, has to be administered as early as possible after the onset of illness.

As mentioned in Chapter 2, when considering the definition of what a virus is, the status of a virus inside the cell must be distinguished from that of a virus outside the cell. In the latter situation, a virus behaves as an inert chemical substance, whereas multiplication and thus 'activity' occurs only when it is inside the cell. As a result of this, antiviral drugs, to be effective, must be able to penetrate into the interior of the cell. In addition, antiviral agents can only be effective by interfering with actively multiplying virus. Therefore, a virus that is in a stage of latency and is not multiplying will not be affected by antiviral drugs. At the present state of technological development, no antiviral drug is able to eliminate a virus from the body if it has the potential for latent infection.

The development of antiviral drugs

Antiviral drugs are designed to interfere with a specific step in the multi-plication cycle of the virus. For example, a drug called amantadine, which is used for influenza A virus infection, prevents the virus from penetrating into the cell and preparing itself for replication. A number of antiviral drugs interfere with the replication of the nucleic acid of the virus, such as in the case of acyclovir and herpes viruses. The agent interferon, pro-duced by the body but also manufactured synthetically for use as a drug, affects viruses at a later stage of replication – the stage when the protein and nucleic acid components of the progeny virus are assembled and released from the infected cell.

The design of antiviral drugs therefore needs carefully to dissect out each of the steps of the viral replication cycle and to exploit any possible biochemical event that is unique or sufficiently different in the virus as compared to the cell for it to be utilized in the development of a poten-tial agent with selective activity. This strategy is referred to as targeted

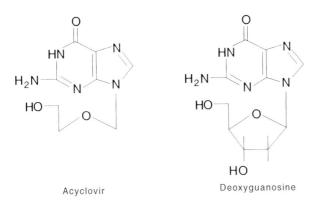

Acyclovir   Deoxyguanosine

Fig. 6.1 Molecular structure of the drug acyclovir and the natural nucleoside deoxyguanosine.

antiviral drug development. The main principle used for the design of these interfering molecules is that of mimicry. Molecules are designed to closely resemble the natural building blocks used by the virus for the manufacture of its structural components. This artificial molecule, often referred to as an analogue of the natural substance, is then taken up by the virus as if it were the natural material itself. The analogue is, however, changed in such a way that it obstructs further biochemical processing, halting the replication cycle at that point and thus preventing the virus from replicating. For example, acyclovir is very similar in structure to the nucleoside deoxyguanosine (Fig. 6.1) which the virus needs to make copies of its DNA. The acyclovir molecule (with its phosphate groups added) is not recognized by the virus as being any different from natural deoxyguanosine, and is incorporated into the growing chain of DNA. However, further elongation of the chain cannot take place onto the acyclovir molecule as would occur with a deoxyguanosine molecule and the growing chain is then terminated at that point. A number of other molecular 'look-alikes' are similarly used as antiviral drugs. The design of these molecules must, of course, be of such a nature as to deceive the virus but not the cell's recognition facilities.

Antiviral drugs are also developed by the more empirical approach of screening natural compounds produced by plants and other biological sources for antiviral activity and, if such a compound is found, its mode of action is then usually subsequently investigated. Widespread screening of literally hundreds of thousands of biological compounds, especially materials produced by fungi and other simple forms of plant life, have been the basis for the development of many successful antibiotics since Alexander

Fleming's accidental discovery of penicillin produced by a contaminating mould in his bacterial cultures in 1928. In recent times hopes for finding useful antiviral agents from plant sources have receded quite considerably and virtually all new useful antiviral drugs have been chemically synthesized.

Occasionally drugs with completely different usages are, quite by accident, found to have antiviral activities. For example, the anti-influenza drug amantadine, which had been used for a number of years for the control of Parkinson's disease, was fortuitously discovered to have a potent inhibitory effect on the replication of the influenza virus.

Therapy of AIDS and HIV infection

There are, essentially, three main elements in the therapy of AIDS. Firstly and foremost, the reduction of mass of virus in the body, that is the viral load, by direct antiviral treatment of the HIV infection itself; secondly, the treatment of the indirect effects of HIV infection, that is the opportunistic infections and the HIV-associated tumours; and thirdly, and today probably the least important, the reconstitution of the immune system which has been so profoundly damaged by the infection.

Antiretroviral drug therapy

The crucial goal of management of HIV infection is the reduction of the burden of the viral load in the body by the administration of drugs which directly inhibit the replication and inactivate HIV (antiretroviral or anti-HIV drugs). The ability to reliably quantify the amount of virus in the blood and other body compartments has clearly demonstrated the direct role that HIV plays in the pathogenesis of HIV disease (see Chapter 3). The viral load test which measures the mass of HIV in the plasma is now a fundamental diagnostic test for the management of HIV infection (see Chapter 5). Antiretroviral drugs that succeed in lowering the viral load in the blood, and by implication in the rest of the body, improve the prognosis of the patient and the opposite is true when these drugs fail to maintain a low or absent plasma viral load. Recent research developments have provided clinicians with a wider range of effective anti-HIV drugs. The modern management of HIV-infected persons now focuses on earlier more aggressive treatment with combinations of anti-HIV drugs to avoid the development of resistance to these drugs by HIV, while monitoring the effectiveness of treatment and the therapeutic response in the patient by measuring the viral load in the plasma and monitoring the CD4 lymphocyte count.

The treatment of the opportunistic infections

Advances and breakthroughs in the prevention and treatment of opportunistic infections have significantly contributed to the improvements in the prognosis of AIDS in the developed world in recent times, as have the developments of anti-HIV drugs. An important example of this has been the treatment of pneumonia caused by the parasite *Pneumocystis carinii*, which is one of the most important causes of death from AIDS in the developed world. The drug pentamidine has been in widespread use for a number decades for the treatment of parasitic diseases such as sleeping sickness. However, it was the recent adaptation of this drug to an aerosol form of administration which was a significant advance in the treatment of AIDS. The drug in this form is inhaled into the respiratory tract, thus bringing it into direct contact with the organism and also avoiding the systemic toxicity which was previously one of the major drawbacks in the use of this agent in treating *Pneumocystis carinii* pneumonia. Aerosolized (nebulized) pentamidine is sometimes recommended for prophylaxis against *Pneumocystis carinii* pneumonia in individuals whose CD4 lymphocyte counts have dropped below 200 per cubic millimetre of blood or who have other signs which make them vulnerable to infections, such as a persistent fever or oral thrush (*Candida*). However, the currently recommended prophylaxis for *Pneumocystic carinii* pneumonia is the antimicrobial agent cotrimoxazole, or alternatively trimethoprim or dapsone. Other advances in the treatment of *Pneumocystis carinii* pneumonia include early usage of high-dose steroids together with aerosolized pentamidine. By far the most important opportunistic infection in the developing world is tuberculosis. It has also assumed major proportions in the inner city populations of many developed countries, particularly the USA. A very worrying development in recent times is the spectre of tuberculosis bacilli that are resistant to many of the drugs used in conventional treatment of this infection. This so-called multi-drug resistant (MDR) tuberculosis is becoming increasingly prevalent in HIV-infected patients and is even posing a risk to health care workers nursing and treating these patients. Prophylaxis against opportunistic tuberculosis with isoniazid is recommended when the CD4 lymphocyte count drops below 300 per cubic millimetre.

Another important opportunistic parasitic infection which commonly causes cerebral disease is toxoplasmosis (caused by *Toxoplasma gondii*). It has recently been shown that standard antimicrobial combinations of sulphadiazine and pyrimethamine can be replaced by an equally effective combination of clindamycin and pyrimethamine, providing clinicians with an important alternative therapeutic option.

The antifungal agents fluconazole and ketaconazole are now being widely used to treat *Candida* as well as for the treatment and prophylaxis of more serious fungal infections such as *Cryptococcus*, which causes severe meningitis, and *Candida* of the oesophagus.

A number of newer antibiotics, especially of the group called macrolides, promise to have greater efficacy against a number of bacterial infections such as *Mycobacterium tuberculosis*, the cause of tuberculosis, and related mycobacteria which cause atypical mycobacterial infections, which in AIDS patients are frequently resistant to conventional antibiotics.

The drug ganciclovir is related to acyclovir, although it does not have the advantage of selective activation as in the case of acyclovir and is consequently considerably more toxic. It is used for the treatment of cytomegalovirus. This virus is one of the commoner causes of serious opportunistic viral infections in AIDS, and is, in addition, resistant to acyclovir. Other drugs, phosphonoformate and cidofovir, are also occasionally used for the treatment of cytomegalovirus.

The treatment of opportunistic infections in AIDS is particularly difficult. The organisms which cause the infections are often unusual organisms which do not respond to the more commonly used antimicrobial agents. In addition, because of the severe suppression of the immune system, there is frequently a high load of these organisms which need to be totally eliminated for recovery to take place, as the host's crippled immune system would probably be unable to carry out the final mopping up of remnant organisms. Resistance to antimicrobial agents frequently develops in these patients because of the high numbers of organisms, their rapid multiplication and the failure to clear up remnant organisms by the immune system, which are then under selective pressure to mutate and develop resistance.

Nevertheless, the advent of a number of newer and highly effective agents, as well as the increasing use of agents for long-term prophylaxis against organisms such as *Pneumocystis carinii*, *Mycobacterium tuberculosis* (which causes tuberculosis), herpes, *Candida* and others has resulted in the significant delaying of the onset of AIDS in patients in the developed world. However, ultimately infections arise which do not respond to treatment and result in the demise of the patient.

Reconstitution and stimulation of the immune system

Therapeutic approaches to the reconstitution of the damaged immune system or stimulation of immune functions have not as yet been successful in patients. A variety of immunostimulatory agents have been evaluated in the past, both experimentally in the laboratory and in patients. Some of these materials have activities confined to the stimulation of the immune system such as dithiocarb (also called immunothiol) and AS-101. Others have combined immunostimulatory as well as antiviral activity, such as ampligen, which consists of a mismatched length of double-stranded RNA. Additional agents in this class include isoprinosine, an agent which is active against RNA viruses and is also an immunostimulant, and interferon which enhances some immune functions in addition to its antiviral activity. There have, however, been few promising indications of therapeutic possibilities with any of these immunostimulatory agents and they have no place in the modern management of the HIV-infected patient.

Alternative therapeutic approaches to reconstitution of the immune system have involved the use of molecules that are physiologically involved in the immune response; for example, transfer factor, which is extracted from the white cells of the blood and derives its name from its ability to transfer elements of the cellular immune response when injected into recipients. Another example is the group of molecules called interleukins, which are messenger molecules produced by some white cells and act as chemical signals to activate other cellular components of the immune system. Materials such as granulocyte-macrophage colony stimulatory factor (GM-CSF) produced by genetic engineering techniques have been evaluated, not only for their effect in restoring immune function but also bone marrow function, which is often depressed either by HIV or by the use of drugs such as AZT. The therapeutic promise of these approaches has, however, not been realized. Paradoxically, there may even be a potential danger that immunostimulatory agents may, in fact, aggravate AIDS by stimulating the production of CD4 lymphocytes and activating them, thus providing additional target cells for the virus to infect and to increase its mass in the body. At the present time attempts to reconstitute the immune system or to stimulate a flagging immune system have little role to play in the management of HIV-infected patients.

Early steps in the development of anti-HIV drugs

In theory HIV should offer a number of targets for the development of drugs that could be selectively active against the virus while sparing the host cell. Foremost amongst these targets is the reverse transcriptase enzyme, on which the virus depends for the replication of its nucleic acid, and which is unique to this family of viruses. Theoretically, therefore, drugs targeting reverse transcriptase should have little or no toxicity to cells. In practice, however, the drugs which are most frequently used in the treatment of AIDS and which act on the reverse transcriptase enzyme of HIV all have significant toxicity.

Worldwide, the research into the development of anti-HIV drugs is unprecedented in its intensity and extent. Immense resources have been devoted both to the empirical screening of biological compounds as well as to the targeted drug design approach.

Empirical screening for anti-HIV drugs

The frustration at the seemingly slow pace of development of drugs to treat HIV infection has provided an enormous impetus to search amongst the huge storehouse of biological compounds found in nature, especially amongst the vast diversity of plant species in the world. The many hundreds of thousands of species of terrestrial plants, which live in almost every conceivable habitat on the planet, from the frozen Arctic wastes to the lush tropical rain forests of continents and remote islands, have come under scrutiny. In addition, an equally varied flora is found in marine plant life, over 100 000 species of fungi and many thousands of species of algae, lichen and related plant life forms. From this virtually inexhaustible supply of biological compounds have come an immense number of substances which are now being screened for antiviral activity in general and for activity against the HIV virus in particular. Automated facilities for large-scale screening of compounds have been established at sophisticated scientific institutions such as the National Institutes of Health in the USA and also by a variety of commercial and pharmaceutical companies. Many of these programmes are each able to screen some 20 000 or more compounds each year. The production of biological compounds for screening is often the result of collaborative investigations with botanical taxonomists who are responsible for the systematic collection of plant species, organic chemists who separate biologically active compounds from plant extracts, and virologists who examine their potential antiviral activities in automated screening and definitive testing procedures. These studies have involved such world renowned botanical collections as those at Kew Gardens in London and have also obtained large amounts of material from many field expeditions to the remotest corners of the globe.

Plant materials and extracts have been used for centuries in traditional medicines by the indigenous inhabitants of all corners of the world. These traditional remedies have been utilized for a variety of medicinal purposes, which have included the treatment of infectious diseases. Indeed, even in orthodox Western medicine, there are many examples of drugs which owe their origins to observations of therapeutic effects when used in traditional medicine. A worldwide call was made by the WHO in February 1989 for investigations to be made of the materials that are used by traditional healers in various parts of the world, to augment current programmes searching for anti-HIV drugs. Unfortunately, despite a number of promising leads and the tantalizing attraction of a relatively inexpensive natural anti-HIV agent, the plant kingdom has still not yielded any materials which could be of any therapeutic value.

Targeted drug design

The direct targeting approach to designing drugs which will specifically interfere with a particular step in the replication process of HIV follows the same principles as with antiviral agents in general. A careful analysis of the replication cycle of the virus is utilized in attempting to design molecules to interfere specifically with each of the steps in the cycle.

Essentially there are two main stages in the replication of HIV – an early stage, where the virus enters the host cell and reaches the point where it is ready to replicate itself, and a late stage of replication of the individual components of the virus and the assembly of these components into progeny virus particles to be released from the cell.

The early stage of replication is composed of a number of individual steps (Fig. 6.2). Firstly, there is the initial attachment of the gp120 glycoprotein protuberance of the virus to its specific CD4 protein receptor site on the cell. This is then followed by fusion of the envelope of the virus to that of the cell membrane (and also, at the same time, cell membranes to each other to produce syncytia). After fusion, the nucleocapsid of the virus (that is, the virus particle minus its envelope) penetrates into the cell and this is then followed by the uncoating step, where the capsid or protein shell is split off to expose the nucleic acid so that it can replicate. The RNA genome of HIV would now need to be reverse transcribed into a complementary DNA form, also referred to as the proviral DNA, which can then integrate into the host cell's chromosomal DNA in order for it to replicate. This reverse transcription is undertaken by the virus-specific reverse transcriptase enzyme which has two separate activities. In the first of these, a DNA strand is manufactured on the RNA template of the virus, a process called DNA polymerization. What is then produced is a hybrid double-stranded molecule consisting of one strand of new DNA and one of the original RNA. The RNA would now need to be digested off for replication to continue, and this is carried out by the second component

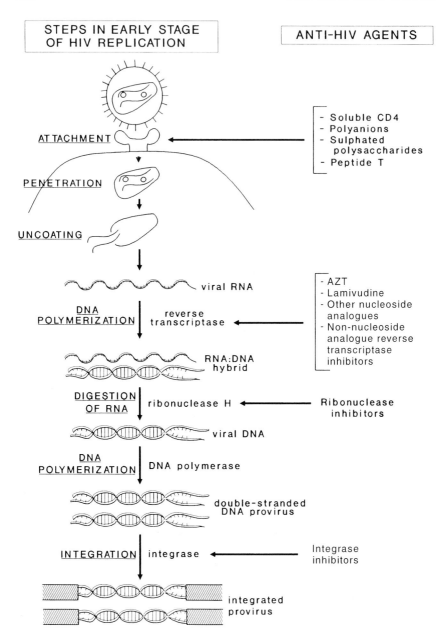

Fig. 6.2 Steps in the early stage of HIV replication, showing sites of activity of anti-HIV drugs.

of the reverse transcriptase enzyme called ribonuclease H. The lone strand of DNA can now itself act as a template for DNA polymerization, to give rise to the double-stranded provirus DNA of HIV which is able to integrate and make copies of itself. Drugs that are effective in interfering with any of these steps in the early stage of replication would be effective in blocking acute HIV infection.

The late stage of HIV replication also consists of a number of separate steps (Fig. 6.3). From this provirus DNA new viral RNA and also messenger RNA are transcribed. The latter then directs the production of protein molecules using the host cell's manufacturing machinery (such as its ribosomes). These protein molecules are, however, not in a state where they can be used for the synthesis of viral particles and they need to undergo further processing. In some cases the functional proteins are actually smaller components of the protein molecules which come off the messenger RNA production line and these larger proteins thus need to be digested into the smaller functional components. This digestion is called proteolysis and the viral enzyme that carries out this function is called protease. Some proteins also need to have additional non-protein molecules added on to them; for example, carbohydrates have to be attached to the envelope proteins to turn them into glycoproteins – a process called glycosylation. The addition of myristic acid to the viral proteins is also required to render them functional, a process called myristylation. Finally, the progeny viral RNA and the processed proteins are assembled into mature viral particles and released from the cell by budding through the cell membrane.

At virtually all of these steps, new drugs have been designed which show activity in the laboratory. Many are already undergoing clinical evaluation and in some cases are presently being used therapeutically.

The initial attachment of the virus' gp120 to the cell's CD4 protein may be blocked by a number of agents. The CD4 protein itself has been manufactured as a soluble protein by genetic engineering techniques. The principle of using soluble CD4 is for it to act as a decoy so that the virus will attach to it in preference to the target cell. Unfortunately, soluble CD4 is unstable in the body and is too rapidly inactivated for it to be clinically useful. To render it more stable CD4 may be fused to immunoglobulins, the CD4-immunoglobulin complex is referred to as an immunoadhesin. The interaction between gp120 and CD4 can also be blocked by highly charged molecules which electrostatically interact with either component of the binding. Thus, a group of molecules called polyanions react mainly with CD4 receptors, while carbohydrate compounds which have sulphur-containing residues attached to them, the sulphated polysaccharides, react

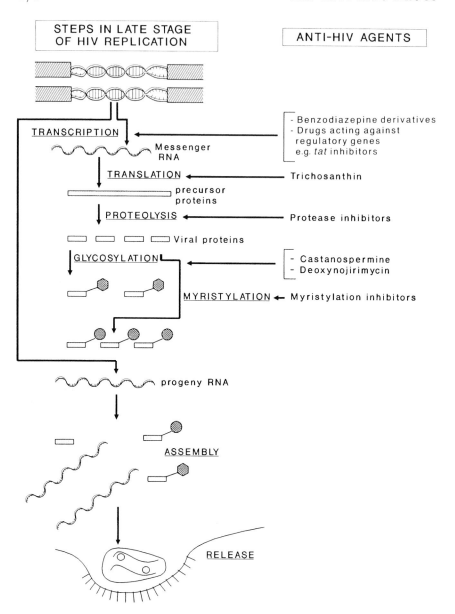

Fig. 6.3 Steps in the late stage of HIV replication, showing sites of activity of anti-HIV drugs.

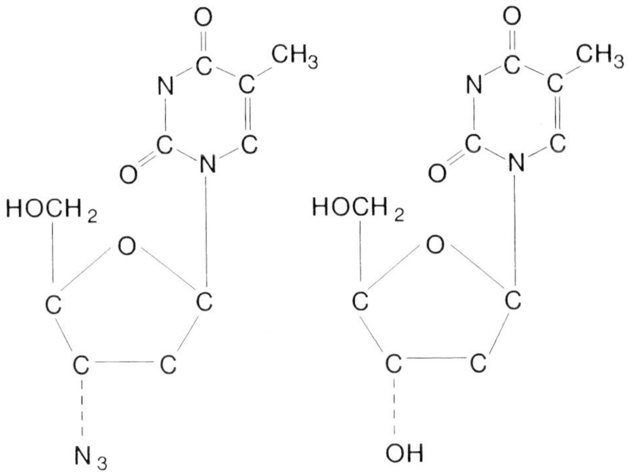

Fig. 6.4 Molecular structure of the drug zidovudine and the natural nucleoside thymidine.

mainly with the gp120 and prevent it from attaching to the cellular receptor site. A number of other decoy molecules have been investigated. One which received a significant amount of publicity, but is now considered to have little or no therapeutic potential, is a substance called peptide T (so called because five of the amino acids of the eight amino acid length polypeptide chain start with the letter T). This compound has considerable similarity to a section of the viral protein gp120 and the peptide T was thought to be effective in preventing viral attachment to CD4.

No potentially useful agents have been designed which interfere with the fusion or penetration steps.

It is the unique step of reverse transcription which has attracted the most attention of drug designers and also yielded the most therapeutically beneficial agents so far. Some of the earliest drugs used in the treatment of AIDS, such as suramin and HPA23, which are no longer used for AIDS therapy, were inhibitors of reverse transcriptase.

The most widely used anti-AIDS drug, azidothymidine (AZT, Retrovir®) is a natural nucleoside analogue consisting of the base thymine attached to a ribose sugar. In fact the molecule is identical to natural thymine-ribose but for the substitution of an azide group (a group of three nitrogen atoms) for a hydroxyl (oxygen-hydrogen group) in the ring structure of the ribose sugar molecule (Fig. 6.4). The reverse transcriptase enzyme of the virus is deceived into incorporating a molecule of AZT in preference to that of the natural nucleoside and the developing DNA chain is then blocked at this point in a similar manner to that of acyclovir and the herpes viruses. As with acyclovir, the AZT molecule is itself inactive and needs to have three phosphate groups added on in succession in order for it to be 'seen' by the reverse transcriptase enzyme and thus be incorporated into the growing nucleic acid chain. The therapeutic successes of AZT as well as its weaknesses in terms of side-effects, and also the ability of the virus to develop resistance to it, have spurred on efforts to develop other drugs with similar molecular configuration. This group of compounds, chemically called the $2',3'$-dideoxynucleosides, have yielded a number of additional valuable therapeutic agents such as dideoxyinosine (ddI), dideoxycytidine (ddC), lamivudine (3TC) and stavudine (d4T). These agents, like AZT, are molecular analogues of natural nucleosides and their modes of action are essentially similar to those of AZT.

In addition to the nucleoside analogue drugs, there are a number of agents that directly target the enzyme reverse transcriptase, such as nevirapine, delavirdine and loviride. These have come to be known as the non-nucleoside reverse transcriptase inhibitors.

Reverse transcriptase is also the target for a remarkable group of compounds called the TIBO (tetrahydroimidazo [4,5,1,-jk]-benzodiazepin-2 (1*H*)-one and-thione) derivatives, which are related to the important group of pharmaceutical substances called the benzodiazepines from which are derived a number of well known sedatives and tranquillizers such as Librium® and Valium®. The mode of action of the TIBO compounds on reverse transcriptase has not been definitively established, but they demonstrate remarkable specificity, being active against HIV-1 only and having little or no activity on HIV-2 or any of the animal immunodeficiency viruses. At present, the limited supply has hampered more extensive investigations of these agents.

More recently another group of benzodiazepine derivatives has been found to have a quite different mode of action. The prototype of this group, code-named RO24-7429, is a potent inhibitor of the *tat* (one of the important regulatory genes of the virus – see Chapter 2) activity of both HIV-1 and HIV-2 viruses as well as SIV. Alternative experimental approaches to inactivating the regulatory genes have involved the use of 'anti-sense' nucleotides. These are short strands of nucleic acid which have a complementary sequence to the gene which is being targeted for inactivation. By attaching to the DNA provirus segment of that gene or else its messenger RNA, an artificial hybrid is created which becomes functionally inactive. Experimental demonstration of viral suppression has been demonstrated, for instance with 'anti-sense' molecules directed against the *rev* gene (see Chapter 2, 'The regulation of HIV').

After the reverse transcriptase enzyme, the next most important target for antiretroviral drug development has been the enzyme protease. This enzyme is responsible for splitting the large precursor proteins that are coded for by the genes of the virus into their smaller structural or enzyme components which are then incorporated into the developing virus during replication. Approximately as many protease inhibitor drugs have been developed as nucleoside analogue reverse transcriptase inhibitors and they are now being used almost as extensively. These agents are commonly used in combination with nucleoside analogue reverse transcriptase inhibitors to maximise the combined antiretroviral effect of each of these classes of drugs and also to reduce the risk of resistance developing because they act on different targets in the virus replication cycle. Some of the more important anti-HIV drugs in this class of agents are saquinavir, ritonavir, indinavir, nelfinavir and VX-478.

The ribonuclease H (RNase H) molecular component of the reverse transcriptase enzyme has also been investigated as a potential target for the development of anti-HIV drugs since the crystallization of the molecule and the characterization of its three-dimensional structure in 1991. This molecule has now been analysed in extraordinary detail by techniques such as X-ray diffraction and the structure determined to a resolution of 2.4 Å (equal to 24 nm, or 24 thousand millionths of a metre).

A number of potential drugs have been investigated which act by inhibiting the production of viral proteins. For example, an inhibitor of viral protein synthesis at the level of ribosomal activity is a natural substance called trichosanthin (also known as compound 'Q' or GLQ223) and is derived from the root tubers of the Chinese cucumber plant *Trichosanthes kirilowii* which has been used extensively in Chinese traditional medicine, for example as an arbortifacient and to treat choriocarcinomas.

The glycosylation of the envelope glycoprotein of the virus is the target of a number of naturally derived anti-HIV compounds. The carbohydrate added to the protein molecule needs to be trimmed in order for the glycoprotein to be functional and substances which interfere with this trimming process are effective in inhibiting viral replication. Two of the most important of these natural compounds are castanospermine, derived from the Australian chestnut *Castanospermum australe* and an antibiotic called deoxynojirimycin.

The process of myristylation has also been investigated as a possible target for antiviral drug development and a number of myristic acid analogues are currently under evaluation.

Finally, a novel direction for targeted drug development which does not involve interfering with the steps of viral replication, but rather exploits the specificity of the viral surface proteins which are found on the outside of infected cells, is to target toxic materials into these cells to destroy them. For example, the linking of the CD4 molecule to a toxic material, such as an exotoxin (toxin secreted by bacteria) from an organism called *Pseudomonas*, produces a hybrid molecule called CD4-PE40 (PE = *Pseudomonas* exotoxin). This molecule will then function like a guided missile to seek out and specifically attach to the HIV-infected cells where viral gp120 protrudes to the outside of the cell membrane. Once the CD4 component has attached to the exposed gp120 it releases its lethal cargo into the cell, thereby destroying only infected cells. Another toxin which has also been coupled onto targeting vehicles is ricin, a compound derived from the castor bean, and one of the most lethal of biological compounds. As an alternate vehicle to CD4 molecules, antibodies directed against gp120 or gp41 are also being investigated.

The status of AIDS drugs

Steps in the evaluation of new drugs

New drugs developed either from deliberate and planned chemical structuring to serve a specific function, or following a more empirical screening approach, are first evaluated in laboratory systems for activity before being investigated in experimental animals for safety and efficacy.

The evaluation of new drugs in humans is taken through three successive phases – phase I, phase II and phase III clinical trials, before licensing as a therapeutic agent can be considered. Phase I evaluation is a preliminary investigation of a new agent for evidence of side-effects and to assess how humans react to the new drug. Phase II examines the dosages needed for distribution of the drug in the body, what levels are achieved in different organs and body fluids and compartments, and also how the drug is eliminated and excreted. The final phase, III, is a definitive evaluation of the efficacy of the agent. In a phase III trial, the performance of the drug in a test population is generally compared to that in a control population receiving a placebo (an inert material disguised to resemble the test drug as closely as possible).

However, in the development of AIDS drugs, in particular, the lengthy evaluation through all three phases required by licensing authorities has often been cut short because of the intense pressures to provide patients with agents that look to be beneficial on preliminary testing, even if they have been incompletely evaluated. For example, in 1986 in the early clinical trials of AZT, 286 patients with AIDS or AIDS-related complex (ARC) were divided equally into a group receiving the agent and a group receiving a placebo. After six months an interim analysis revealed a highly significant reduction in mortality in the group receiving AZT (one death compared to 19 deaths in the placebo group). These findings led to the abandonment of the placebo group and all patients involved in the trial were then provided with AZT treatment. The licensure of AZT was approved even though a full evaluation was not completed. Accelerated licensing of other anti-HIV drugs has also taken place on a similar compassionate basis – so-called 'fast-track' licensing.

'Unlicensed' anti-AIDS agents

A large repertoire of drugs and biological compounds are currently under evaluation or being used for the treatment of AIDS, but are not, at present, licensed for clinical usage in developed countries. These include chemical substances fresh from the planning stage of targeted drug design programmes and shown in the laboratory to block HIV infection, or compounds extracted from plant materials and shown in cell culture to have anti-HIV activity, or other drugs or materials which, quite incidentally, have been shown to have anti-HIV activity.

There are a number of materials which have been under evaluation for some years in both phase I and phase II trials but have still not been found to be adequately effective for them to be licensed for general clinical usage. Many of the experimental materials mentioned above fall into this group. Dextran sulphate is one of the most widely used of these compounds and was originally manufactured on a large scale by the Japanese pharmaceutical industry and is widely used in Japan for a number of other conditions. Large amounts of material were imported illegally into the USA by community-based gay organizations and buyers groups for use by AIDS patients. There is still substantial non-medically supervised usage of this substance in spite of some quite marked side-effects such as vomiting, diarrhoea and abdominal discomfort. Trichosanthin (compound Q) is another example of a substance still undergoing such evaluation as well as hypericin, a compound derived from the St John's wort (*Hypericum* sp.) and used commonly in herbal medicine and shown to have strong antiretroviral activity.

On occasion, considerable excitement is generated by the 'advent' of a new potential anti-HIV agent and frequently extravagant but premature claims are made for it. Many of these materials have been subject to phase

I and some even phase II trials, but have not yet been found to have a significant therapeutic benefit. Into this category are a number of immuno-stimulatory agents, such as ampligen, AS-101, isoprinosine and dithiocarb. Other materials that have come and gone include fusidic acid, which is an antimicrobial agent used to treat, for example, urinary tract infections. This agent, similar to the bile salts of the body, has a detergent activity which can affect the membrane of viruses such as HIV. Another compound having an effect on viral membranes, which enjoyed a heyday of popu-larity especially in non-medically supervised therapy, was AL 721. This mixture of lipids derived from egg yolks, extracts cholesterol from the lipid membranes of cells and viruses and the resulting perturbation of mem-brane function was thought to affect the virus' ability to attach to cells.

Many materials are held to have anti-HIV activity on the basis of non-scientifically based or proven reasons and are obtained and utilized by AIDS patients. Often these materials are made in backyard laboratories or smuggled into countries like the USA from abroad. Underground buying networks have sprung up and so-called 'guerilla clinics' have been estab-lished to treat AIDS patients outside the medical profession. The recurrent disappointments arising from premature claims of drug 'breakthroughs' which do not materialize have often led to increasing despair and despon-dency amongst patients and their families, and this, in turn, further exacer-bates their feelings of distrust of the medical profession. The wedge has been further widened by the anger at the perceived manner in which the clinical trials of potential agents are being carried out with relatively low numbers and over frustratingly long periods of time. It is precisely this impatience which led to the political pressure for the accelerated compas-sionate licensing of anti-HIV drugs. Frequently AIDS patients, even though they may be part of a medically supervised clinical trial, will also secretly take 'underground' medications which may confuse and obfuscate the inter-pretation of clinical findings.

Occasionally these medications may be harmful to the patient. For exam-ple, the uncontrolled stimulation of immune cells by immunostimulatory preparations, if they do work, may aggravate HIV infection by providing the virus with additional activated lymphocytes to infect. Some of these materials may interact negatively with orthodox antiviral agents and their activities may be antagonistic to each other, for example, dextran sulphate and CD4. Lastly, these patients are particularly vulnerable to being exploited by criminals who prey on the desperate and they can ill-afford the loss of their meagre financial resources.

In recent times anti-HIV therapy has made great strides forward and has now reached the stage where judicious usage of combinations of licensed drugs can significantly improve the quality of life, prolong the asymptomatic period and extend survival. Scientific advances have provided clinicians with powerful tools to drastically reduce the load of virus in the body and thereby reduce the damage done to the immune system. Furthermore, diagnostic tests such as the plasma viral load assay provide the clinician with a precise indication of how successful the therapy is or alternately if the drug or drugs are failing as well as giving a good idea of the outlook for the patient. As a result of this, interest in most of the earlier unproven remedies mentioned above has dropped or even disappeared. Effective, albeit not optimal, anti-HIV drugs are now available – the major stumbling block now is cost.

Zidovudine (AZT)

History and development of the drug

The molecule zidovudine was first synthesized by Horwitz in 1964 and was shown soon afterwards to have activity directed against retroviruses responsible for leukaemias and related malignancies in experimental mice, although no possible clinical usefulness in humans was recognized at that stage. In October 1985 its anti-HIV activity was first described by Mitsuya and colleagues at the National Cancer Institute, a part of the National Institutes of Health, in the USA. In the same year, the pharmaceutical company Burroughs Wellcome (now part of Glaxo-Wellcome), which had sent a number of nucleoside analogues, including AZT, to the National Cancer Institute for screening, won an exclusive patent on the drug and received from the Institute a supply of the starting base thymine. Initially, the difficulty in obtaining supplies of thymine, which is extracted from herring sperm, together with the 26 steps and several months of production of the final product, as well as the 'many millions of dollars' spent on research, resulted in the drug being very expensive. When first introduced into the market place, each capsule cost US $3 and the average annual cost of treatment was about $10 000. However, economies of scale and increased availability of thymine enabled the price to be cut by two thirds to $1.20 per capsule with an annual cost of treatment of about $2000 – $3000. (More recently a coalition of AIDS patients has brought a lawsuit against the company challenging its patent on the basis that the discovery of the anti-HIV activity of AZT was made by Mitsuya and the National Cancer Institute rather than the pharmaceutical company. A successful outcome would mean that AZT would become public property which could

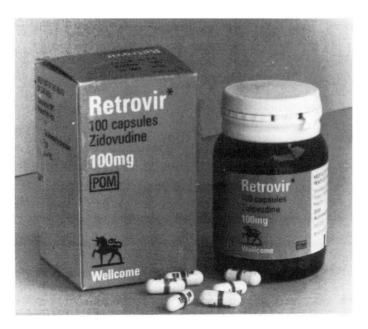

Fig. 6.5 Retrovir (zidovudine)

be produced by generic drug manufacturers at a fraction of the cost. The patent is already being challenged in Canada by two pharmaceutical companies who have claimed to be able to produce AZT as cheaply as 50 cents a capsule.)

Therapeutic usage of zidovudine (AZT)

AZT (Fig. 6.5) is still used extensively in the treatment of AIDS and HIV infection throughout the world. There is little question about the general therapeutic efficacy of the drug. Major improvements, especially in neurological manifestations, reduction in the severity and frequency of opportunistic infections and a significant enhancement of the quality of life, have been consistently demonstrated in symptomatic patients treated with AZT. However, there are two major limitations to the usage of AZT on its own – resistance and toxicity. If AZT is used as the sole anti-HIV drug (monotherapy) failure is inevitable due to the development of resistance by the HIV virus – usually within six months.

In addition, the majority of patients on long-term therapy will experience major toxicity effects of the agent which, in many cases, will force the patients to stop therapy. The most important toxic effect is the suppression of the bone marrow due to the drug inhibiting the replication of the precursor cells in the bloodstream, which are housed in the bone marrow. These precursor cells need to multiply rapidly to continue replenishing the cells of the bloodstream as they die off. More than half of all patients on long-term therapy with AZT will require blood transfusions to replenish their blood cells because of the suppression of the bone marrow. Another significant side-effect is damage to muscle (myopathy), including heart muscle. Myopathy is also a fairly common manifestation of HIV infection itself and is also seen in untreated patients. Nausea, vomiting and diarrhoea are common, but less serious, side-effects, and are often temporary.

Because of the problems of resistance and toxicity, AZT monotherapy is not recommended for long-term therapy. Combination therapy either with another nucleoside analogue reverse transcriptase inhibitor (often lamivudine) or preferably triple therapy (with the addition of a protease inhibitor such as indinavir) is the current choice of anti-HIV therapy. This reduces the chance of development of resistance because the virus would need to mutate at a number of different sites in order for it to develop resistance to a multitude of drugs. Combination therapy also allows for lower doses to be used of, for example, AZT and thereby decreases the incidence and severity of the side-effects. AZT monotherapy still does have a role in short-term therapy as resistance is very unlikely to develop, as for example in treatment of HIV-infected mothers to prevent transmission to the infant or, in some cases, for post-exposure prophylaxis, as will be discussed below.

Modern approaches to anti-HIV therapy

Current approaches to anti-HIV therapy have been greatly influenced by the results of recent studies of the pathogenesis of HIV infection and specifically the dramatic revelation of the vast turnover of virus as well as lymphocytes which occur in the body even in the clinically silent phase of the infection (see Chapter 3). The enormity of this turnover, which has been demonstrated by viral load studies, is truly staggering – up to ten billion or more new HIV virus particles produced daily and up to two billion CD4 lymphocytes destroyed every day. This has underscored the importance of aggressively treating with as powerful a combination of anti-HIV drugs at as early a stage as possible before the immune system is too extensively damaged by this huge onslaught by the virus. These studies have also emphasized the importance of measuring the amount of virus in the plasma by viral load assays to assess the response to therapy. The level of virus in the plasma accurately reflects the total burden of the virus in the body, most of which is actually resident in the lymphoid tissue. Current therapy is therefore based on early treatment with a combination of three drugs and regular monitoring of the viral load in the plasma.

There have been some reservations concerning the immediate commencement of therapy with a triple drug combination, for example from the British HIV Association. The latter body, in contrast to the American recommendations, have advised deferring the commencement of therapy until laboratory markers have indicated that a deterioration in immune function has occurred and the viral load in plasma has started to climb. They also advise commencing therapy with a combination of two nucleoside analogues rather than a triple drug combination. These more cautionary and conservative recommendations are grounded on concerns of the difficulties that patients often have in complying with instructions to take a large number of pills at set times in the day, some of which may have to be taken with food and others on an empty stomach, and yet others require specific dietary modifications such as a fat-free diet. Another concern is that if the patient needs to change drugs, either because the virus becomes resistant or alternatively if toxicity develops, early treatment with three drugs could limit the choices of alternate drugs to change to. In this respect it is crucial for the doctor to discuss the implications of lifelong treatment with very expensive drugs which do have significant to serious side-effects, which have inconvenient and intrusive requirements and which demand rigid and consistent adherence to prescribed regimens of treatment. If compliance with therapy is inadequate this could well lead to the virus 'breaking through' and developing resistance.

Initiating therapy

The most common triple drug combination for commencing therapy is AZT together with lamivudine and the protease inhibitor indinavir. The dosage of AZT has considerably reduced in comparison to that which is used for monotherapy, i.e. either 500 mg per day (a 100 mg capsule five times per day) or 600 mg per day (a 200 mg capsule three times per day). The dose of lamivudine is 150 mg twice a day and that of indinavir 800 mg three times per day. Therapy with multiple drug combinations has now come to be known as HAART (highly active antiretroviral therapy).

A number of clinical trials have investigated a variety of other combinations which have also proved effective. These include combinations with other members of the same class of anti-HIV drugs or alternately substituting a non-nucleoside reverse transcriptase inhibitor or two protease inhibitors with one nucleoside analogue.

Changing therapy

Patients put onto a triple drug regimen should be regularly monitored for viral load levels in the plasma as well as CD4 lymphocyte counts and laboratory evidence of bone marrow or liver toxicity. The regimen may need to be changed if evidence develops of drug failure as indicated by an increasing level of viral load in the plasma, a drop in the CD4 lymphocyte count or the onset of signs and symptoms of clinical disease. Alternatively, the regimen will need to be changed if intolerable toxicity develops or if the patient finds difficulty in compliance with the regimen for a particular drug combination. When changing drugs it is often necessary to change two or three of the drugs in the combination. Fortunately there are now a number of alternatives in each class of drug to choose from.

Costs

There have been very positive and gratifying new drug developments to the point where HIV therapy has at last reached a stage where meaningful and significant therapeutic responses are regularly attainable. Unfortunately, however, the cost of these agents coupled with the high cost of plasma load monitoring, has put this kind of therapy well beyond the reach of the great majority of HIV-infected persons. Nevertheless, in developed countries, the high cost of antiretroviral therapy needs to be seen in the context of the costs saved by delaying hospitalization and preventing opportunistic infections as well as keeping productive young people economically active in the workplace.

There are two special circumstances where a short course of antiretroviral therapy may be contemplated. One of these involves the use of antiretroviral drugs for prophylaxis against HIV infection in non-infected individuals exposed to infection. This situation has been most frequently encountered in the case of health care workers exposed to the virus when injured by a needle or sharp instrument contaminated with blood from an infected patient. It also occasionally arises following other exposures, such as sexual exposure, for example in incidents such as rape by an assailant of known or unknown HIV status. The scientific basis for post-exposure AZT prophylaxis rests, to a large extent, on some experimental animal work reported in 1986, which demonstrated that AZT protected mice from infection with a retrovirus called the Rauscher murine leukaemia virus, and also cats from feline leukaemia virus. In the former case, the drug was effective when administered within four hours after exposure and, in the latter, within one hour after exposure. Two years later, the efficacy of post-exposure AZT prophylaxis was corroborated with HIV in experiments using the so-called SCID-hu mouse model (mice whose own immune systems are congenitally non-functional but who have had immune function restored by the transplantation of cells from the human immune system). However, a succession of experimental animal models, including SIV transmission in primates, have failed to demonstrate any protective efficacy of prophylactic AZT. It is, however, very doubtful whether any meaningful extrapolation of these animal experiments can be made to the situation of HIV transmission to humans, either to prove or to disprove the efficacy of prophylactic AZT. Not only are the biological systems quite different, but the artificially high doses used in these experiments are quite disproportionate to the natural situation.

In the late 1980s a prospective trial of prophylactic AZT was attempted, but had to be terminated in 1989 because an evaluation of the efficacy would have been impossible due to the low rate of infection following a needle-stick incident (0.3%) as well as difficulties in enrolling individuals who had been exposed to infection into the placebo control group. To date eight cases have been reported in health care workers where prophylactic AZT administration failed to prevent infection in individuals who had penetrating injuries involving infected blood.

Up until 1996 recommendations for AZT prophylaxis following possible exposure to HIV was not based on very definite scientific evidence that it would be effective. Public health bodies such as the CDC did not, therefore, consider AZT prophylaxis as 'a necessary component of post-exposure management'. Their recommendations changed, however, in 1996 following the publication of a retrospective study of some 31 health care workers in the USA, UK and France who had become infected with HIV as a result of occupational exposure. When this group was compared to a control group of health care workers who also sustained penetrating injuries with HIV-contaminated blood but who had not become infected, it became apparent that the taking of AZT for prophylaxis reduced the risk of HIV transmission by 79%. Ideally one would have liked the reassurance of a prospective trial to be convinced of the effectiveness of post-exposure prophylaxis. Nevertheless, this study together with mounting evidence of the efficacy of treatment and of prophylaxis, for example in pregnant mothers, now convinced various public health bodies such as the CDC to change their recommendations in favour of post-exposure prophylaxis.

Recommendations to health care workers who have had a penetrating injury with HIV-infected body fluids are based on two considerations –

the volume of the contaminating blood which could have been transferred to the health care worker and the expected level of virus in the blood. The volume of contaminated blood transferred will depend on the depth of the injury, the kind of needle or instrument (hollow injection type needle or solid suture type needle), or, the lowest risk, a splash onto mucous membrane. The level of virus in the blood will be higher in the very early stage of infection (that is soon after infection) and at the latter stages, especially the terminal phase of the illness. Using these two criteria, post-exposure prophylaxis will either be offered (for relatively low-risk situations), recommended (for moderate-risk situations), or strongly encouraged (for high-risk situations). Treatment should be commenced as soon as possible, but at least within 24 hours, or some authorities feel 72 is more reasonable. The present recommendations are for a combination of antiretroviral drugs rather than AZT alone and usually the combination of AZT and lamivudine is used. If the source patient, that is the patient from whom the contaminating blood came, had been on AZT or other antiretroviral therapy for six months or more, then a third antiretroviral, usually the protease inhibitor indinavir, is also added because of the concern about resistance. This therapy should be maintained for four weeks. Blood specimens taken at six weeks and six months are then tested for HIV antibodies and if negative the exposed health care worker can be reassured that transmission of HIV infection had not occurred. The efficacy of post-exposure prophylaxis following other exposures, for example, sexual exposure, has not yet been defined. Nevertheless, the same principles of post-exposure prophylaxis are used, for example following rape or sexual assault.

The other situation where short-term AZT therapy has been shown to be an effective intervention is treatment of pregnant mothers to prevent transmission to the infant. In a landmark study published in 1994 (Aids Clinical Trial Group, ACTG 076), AZT treatment of pregnant mothers between 14 and 34 weeks of gestation was shown to reduce the rate of transmission to the infant by 67.5%. A number of investigations with varying dosages and durations of treatment of the mother at various stages of pregnancy as well as treatment of the newborn infant are being carried out. Short-term AZT therapy in pregnancy, which is relatively inexpensive, offers the first possibility of successful intervention possibility in the developing world where infection of infants is such a considerable problem.

The potential for a drug cure of AIDS

The outlook for the therapy of HIV infection has markedly improved over the past few years. The range of effective anti-HIV drugs has been considerably widened and, in particular, the advent of newer drugs which attach the reverse transcriptase and protease enzymes of the virus have substantially improved the armamentarium available to the practising physician. Early and aggressive therapy with a triple combination of drugs acting at different sites on the virus is now able, in the majority of patients, to drastically reduce the load of virus in the body and this can be precisely measured by newer viral load diagnostic tests. The wide variety of drugs offers doctors a number of alternatives should patients be unable to continue with a particular regimen, or if particular drugs fail to overcome the virus because of resistance. Further studies have demonstrated that not only is there a dramatic reduction in plasma viral load to the point where it is no longer detectable by sensitive PCR tests, but, in addition, there also appears to be a corresponding elimination of virus in the lymphoid tissue, the main sanctuary of the virus, and even a disappearance of virus trapped on the surface of the follicular dendritic cells in the lymph glands. Some researchers have now been emboldened to develop mathematical models which predict that persistent suppression of the virus with this kind of combination therapy could totally eradicate the virus from the body in 2.3 to 3.1 years of treatment. The consensus of opinion, however, believes that the means still do not exist to totally eradicate the virus in its latent form in the cell and that viral embers remaining behind in various sanctuary sites, such as the brain, still carry the potential of rekindling infection after long-term treatment. Nevertheless, the outlook for anti-HIV therapy has improved dramatically in recent years for those who are in a position to afford it. Unfortunately, for the great majority of persons who are in need of anti-HIV therapy, these advances are largely academic. The real challenge for the future will be to focus newer therapeutic advances on costs as well as effectiveness – only then will there be meaningful progress globally in the treatment of HIV infection.

7

The quest for the HIV vaccine

Existing options for the control of HIV infection appear to have limited chances of reversing, let alone curbing, the AIDS epidemic. Efforts at educating populations at large to transform centuries-old practices of intimate behaviour do not seem likely to meet with major and sustained successes. Even in well-motivated and empowered groups, such as populations of homosexual men in the USA, evidence of reversion to high-risk behaviour is now being reported. Drug therapy of HIV infection has, to date, produced clinically beneficial but expensive toxic and non-curative agents. As discussed in the previous chapter, there are, at least in the immediate future, no prospects of designing a drug able to eradicate persistent infections from the body. Thus, on an epidemiological level at least, antiviral drugs hold no promise for curbing the expansion of the epidemic.

It is, therefore, not surprising that efforts of an unprecedented intensity have been focused on the development of a vaccine to prevent HIV infection. The power of the vaccine to eradicate, to eliminate, to control and to modify infectious diseases is indeed awesome. Smallpox, that scourge of Europe in the Middle Ages, which has affected human history more profoundly than war and was largely responsible, together with measles, for the fall of the Roman Empire and the conquest of the New World, was declared as eradicated from the planet on 26 October 1977, some 200 years after the vaccine was first used by Edward Jenner. Poliomyelitis, another viral infection which devastated humanity in the first half of this century, is now close to being extinguished by a highly effective vaccine. Also diphtheria, whooping cough, measles, rubella and mumps have all been dramatically reduced and, in some countries, even eliminated, by the widespread use of effective vaccines.

LIVERPOOL JOHN MOORES UNIVERSITY
LEARNING SERVICES

The vaccines developed in past decades were highly effective, safe, cheap and easy to administer. In developed countries, widespread routine vaccination has achieved remarkable success in terms of coverage with its resultant effects on the prevalence of the infection. In countries such as the USA, routine vaccination has been indirectly compulsory by being made a condition of entry for children into schools. In the developing world – as a result of co-ordinated campaigns such as those by the WHO, specifically its Expanded Programme on Immunization (EPI) – vast strides have been taken in increasing the distribution and administration of vaccine since the eradication of smallpox. Thus, by 1991, 80% of the world's children were immunized against the six vaccine-preventable diseases that form the target of the EPI programme, tuberculosis, measles, diphtheria, whooping cough, tetanus and poliomyelitis. The availability of a cheap, safe and effective vaccine is therefore only the first step in controlling the infection. The adequate and sustained distribution of this vaccine is the final goal.

These vaccines, which have been so effective in controlling infection, have all been relatively easy to design and produce. Also, the diseases for which they are effective have, in the main, been acute illnesses, with a defined immune response by the body which is effective both for recovery from the disease and for protection from re-infection. The viruses are also usually of a single, unchanging antigenic type and the viral vaccines were produced simply by killing or inactivating the viruses with chemicals or heat, or mutating them into vaccine strains by 'hit and miss' empirical processes. It is, indeed, for a number of reasons fortunate that the AIDS epidemic was born into the last two decades of the century when not only diagnostic capabilities but also technologies for future vaccine development are now so much more advanced. Nevertheless, the problems in designing a vaccine for a virus which is so highly variable and so efficient in its ability to escape the immune response of the host present a unique challenge of daunting complexity. Before considering these difficulties and the progress which has been achieved so far, it would be as well to examine some general aspects of the design of viral vaccines.

The development of viral vaccines

The definition and principles of vaccines

A broad definition of a vaccine is that of a material which is administered to an individual to stimulate their immune system to give protection from infection with a specific micro-organism. As the immune system is specifically activated by the protein components of the organism, the same immune response can also be achieved by administering only the relevant proteins of the organism. Thus, for viral vaccines purified proteins are used which can be produced by genetic engineering technologies, as in the case of the hepatitis B vaccine, or the whole virus particle may be used after it has been 'killed' or inactivated by chemicals or heat as, for example, with influenza vaccine, rabies vaccine and the inactivated poliomyelitis vaccine. A vaccine composed of the antigenic proteins alone is referred to as a sub-unit vaccine and that composed of the whole virus particle which has been inactivated or 'killed', as an inactivated or killed virus vaccine. Naturally there is no danger that these kinds of vaccines are able to produce the diseases associated with that virus.

An alternative approach to making viral vaccines is to keep the virus alive and able to replicate in the host. These live viral vaccines are pro-duced by genetically altering the natural virus, which is referred to as the wild-type virus (the virus found in the 'wild', that is, in nature), to produce a vaccine virus that has lost its ability to cause disease while still retaining the same potential to stimulate the host's immune system. This genetically changed vaccine virus strain differs from the wild-type strain by a varying number of mutations. For example, the live poliomyelitis vaccine strains differ from their wild-type counterparts by 10–56 mutations. This process of reducing the pathogenic potential of wild-type virus to produce a vac-cine virus is called attenuation, and these vaccines are often referred to as live attenuated vaccines. All live vaccines in routine use today have been attenuated by a 'hit and miss' empirical process of growing wild-type virus in tissue culture through numerous passages. During this procedure the wild-type virus progressively accumulates mutations which make it more adapted to growth in cell culture while, at the same time, it loses its ability to cause disease in its natural host. Eventually, usually after a few hundred passages through cell culture, a strain is arrived at which will still be able to multiply in its natural host and stimulate the immune system in a sim-ilar way to the wild-type virus but will now virtually have lost its disease-producing potential. On very rare occasions live vaccine strains may still produce disease; for example, a measles-like illness may occur in some children from the measles vaccine, or paralytic poliomyelitis may take place as a very rare complication (about one in every two to three million doses of vaccine) due to the vaccine strain mutating back to the virulent form. With advances in science and technology, new live vaccines may well, in the future, be more scientifically produced by purposefully engineering pre-determined mutations for attenuation into the wild-type strain to produce a more predictably and reliably attenuated vaccine virus.

LIVERPOOL
JOHN MOORES UNIVERSITY
AVRIL ROBARTS LRC
TEL. 0151 231 4022

Finally, one of the oldest forms of vaccination, from which the word vaccination is derived (vacca = cow), is the use of animal viruses that are antigenically sufficiently similar to produce protective immunity, but lack the potential to produce disease in humans. Historically the first successful human vaccine, developed by Edward Jenner in 1798, used a virus which produced pox in cows as a vaccine against smallpox in humans. This so-called Jennerian approach to vaccination has recently again been given consideration for some other human virus vaccines; for example, against rotavirus, the major causal agent of gastroenteritis in infants.

Viral vaccines and their usage in Man

All subunit and inactivated viral vaccines presently in use are administered by injection. The material, being foreign to the body, is ingested by the antigen-presenting cells, macrophages and dendritic cells, at the site of the injection and 'presented' to the immune system for the latter to develop a specific immune response. Protection against infection is largely due to the IgG antibodies in the person's bloodstream.

The live attenuated vaccines are also mostly administered by injection, such as the measles, mumps, rubella and yellow fever vaccines, or they may be given via the same route as the natural infection, for example live poliomyelitis vaccine is given by mouth. When given by injection, the live virus particles are also ingested by antigen-presenting cells, but the live vaccine virus undergoes cycles of replication, thus providing a stronger stimulation of the immune system than in the case of the inactivated vaccines. The immunity is, therefore, generally of greater duration and often may be life-long even after a single dose of vaccine, and resembles the quality of immunity following a natural infection. It is similarly mainly due to IgG in the blood. In addition, however, live vaccines given by the natural route, for example oral poliomyelitis vaccine, multiply in the surface epithelium, in this case the gut, as is the case with wild-type virus in a natural infection. As a result, the local immune system of the gut is strongly stimulated in addition to the general immune system of the body, resulting in very effective local immunity in the gut (due to IgA antibodies) as well as the IgG antibodies produced in the bloodstream.

A very important component of the immune system which ensures that vaccines have long-term effectiveness is its memory function. The memory cells of the immune system operate much like the back-up system of a computer. All encounters with antigens are registered by the memory of the immune system in these cells, so that when the same antigen is experienced again the immune response is very much quicker and will rapidly eliminate the infectious organism even before it has a chance to cause any symptoms, and as a result the patient is usually unaware of the re-infection. Nevertheless, the limited amount of replication that does take place may still be sufficient to give the immune system a boost. In nature the long-lasting effect of immunity which is seen following infection or vaccination with a live virus vaccine is, in many cases, probably due to recurrent bouts of re-infection. With each one there is an accelerated immune response, due to the memory cells, which eliminates the invading organism before the patient is aware of having been re-infected. The resultant boosting of the immune response thus perpetuates the immune system's protection against the organism.

In the final analysis, the effectiveness of a vaccine is only relative to the quality of the immune response on the one hand, and the dose of invading organisms on the other. In many situations, even vaccines that produce very good immunity may be overwhelmed by vast numbers of invading organisms and a 'breakthrough' infection may result. This is not uncommonly seen; for example, with measles vaccination in developing countries where 'breakthrough' infections occur not uncommonly in the overcrowded conditions of socio-economically deprived communities, even though the vaccine itself usually provides excellent immunity.

Future viral vaccine research directions

The development of new viral vaccines is a branch of medical research in which there is intense activity in universities, research institutions and in the pharmaceutical and biotechnology industries. This new science is referred to as vaccinology. However, it must be emphasized that it is the classic and empirically constructed viral vaccines of the previous generation that eradicated smallpox from the globe and are targeted to eradicate poliomyelitis by the end of the century; they have also drastically reduced the incidence of a number of viral infections such as measles, mumps and rubella in the developed world. The shortfall that must be overcome before diseases such as measles can be eradicated is due far more to deficiencies in the delivery of the vaccine, especially in the developing world, than to any inadequacies in what are really very effective, safe and cheap vaccines.

Many avenues of vaccinology research are currently being pursued. In some cases research is devoted to the development of vaccines for infections where no vaccines exist at present; for example, respiratory syncytial virus (the major cause of infantile pneumonia), hepatitis C virus and dengue virus (a major viral disease of the tropics). In other cases, vaccine research is involved in improvements of the quality of existing vaccines.

Antigenic proteins for use as subunit vaccines may now be chemically synthesized in the laboratory or on an industrial scale. They may also be made by genetic engineering technologies where the gene for a particular protein is spliced into the chromosome of a bacterial, yeast or mammalian cell, and these cells are then used as factories to make that particular protein. Viral protein genes may also be spliced into the genome of another virus which can then infect its own specific host, for example an insect or plant, and the latter can be cultivated together with the virus carrying the spliced-in gene. For example, the insect virus baculovirus has been demonstrated to be a very exuberant producer of proteins from foreign genes spliced into it. The simplest and most productive way of growing this virus is to infect its natural host, the caterpillar, which can in turn be grown to great profusion under controlled climatic conditions and ample supplies of leafy vegetation. The desired protein can then be extracted from the caterpillar in large amounts and in a particularly purified form, and there is the added benefit that the insect viruses and insect protein are unlikely to cause side-effects in any human vaccine.

The genetic engineering process of splicing a foreign gene into the chromosome of a host cell or host virus is referred to as recombination, because the foreign gene is recombined with the host genome. The technology is called recombinant technology and the resulting proteins which are produced are referred to as recombinant proteins. Using these new recombinant production methods for the specific antigens that are needed for vaccines, it is conceivable that a future vaccine may consist of a single dose of material containing a compendium of all the necessary antigens produced by these genetic engineering or synthetic chemical techniques, which are then attached to a 'carrier' molecule. Research into suitable 'carrier' molecules has also been actively searching for safe materials which are effective in enhancing the immune response to specific antigens.

A different but equally exciting avenue of vaccine research utilizes recombinant techniques to splice the desired protein genes into viruses which have already proven themselves to be effective vaccines and to use these 'carrier' viruses to vaccinate against the recombinant proteins from other viruses. For example, the vaccinia virus (the virus strain used as a vaccine against smallpox) is now being widely explored as a carrier of genes for antigenic proteins to a variety of organisms including HIV. Unfortunately vaccinia virus has caused some significant and even serious side-effects in the past and a related pox virus which infects canaries, the canarypox virus, is being intensively investigated as a possible human vaccine carrier for a number of infectious diseases. Similar studies have also involved the poliomyelitis vaccine virus as well as a number of other common, non-pathogenic viruses such as adenovirus.

Viral vaccine research has also examined ways of replacing the haphazard way of attenuating live vaccines with a more planned and predetermined engineering of the relevant mutations. Techniques have also been developed to take some genes from non-pathogenic variants of viruses and recombine them with the relevant genes for protective antigens taken from the pathogenic wild-type virus to produce new vaccine strains. In a similar way, the construction of an artificial chimera from two different viruses is now feasible, thus enabling a single vaccine virus to immunize simultaneously against a number of different pathogenic organisms.

One of the most exciting of the new vaccine developments has been the advent of DNA vaccines. Quite by accident it was noted that naked DNA containing the gene coding for a particular antigen could be used as a vaccine to elicit an immune response against that antigen. Naked DNA injected into the muscle of an experimental animal is taken up by the muscle cells (later also shown to be as effective if injected into the skin) and the DNA then produces the relevant antigen in those cells, which in turn stimulate an immune response. This immune response is highly protective and both antibody and cellular immunity are produced. A number of DNA vaccines against important human pathogens, including HIV, have been successfully evaluated in experimental animals. These vaccines show exceptional promise for future human vaccine development because of the effectiveness of the immune response they elicit, both humoral and cellular, the durability of the immune response (because of the continual production of antigen by the DNA) and the breadth of the immune response. However, because of safety concerns and especially the need to be reassured that the incorporated DNA carries no possible risk of inducing malignant changes in cells, these vaccines have not yet undergone trials in humans.

All of these research technologies have also been investigated in relation to the development of an HIV vaccine. Many of them have been successful at a laboratory level, that is they have produced copious amounts of the relevant gp120 antigen (or its precursor protein gp160) which is needed to elicit protective antibodies. Many have also been effective in producing neutralizing antibodies in experimental animals and some are being used for phase I and phase II clinical trials. The final development of an effective HIV vaccine is, however, a task which is vastly more difficult than was the development of the other vaccines presently available.

Obstacles to the development of HIV vaccines

The prevailing mood regarding the development of an HIV vaccine was decidedly pessimistic up to the end of the 1980s. The chances of reaching the goal of an effective and safe vaccine was widely held to be 'near hopeless'. There were three main groups of reasons for this despondency:

Virological difficulties

It was feared that the properties of the virus and the features of the relationship between itself and its host would make an effective HIV vaccine impossible to design. Thus, the virus seems to possess properties enabling it to escape from the immune system either by constantly changing itself antigenically or by making itself 'invisible' to the immune system, or by making itself inaccessible to the immune response. There appeared, therefore, to be little value in stimulating the immune system with a vaccine which would be unable to effectively deal with the virus. To make matters worse there are also possible factors in the interaction between the virus and its host which could make a vaccine, in theory at least, do more harm than good. Each of these obstacles can now be examined in somewhat more detail.

One of the cardinal features of the HIV virus which enables it to escape from the host's immune response is its variability. The variability is seen especially in that portion of the virus which is crucial to its attachment to the CD4 receptor site of the cell, namely the third variable segment (V3 loop) of the gp120 envelope glycoprotein. Variability is seen even with different strains called quasispecies, being generated and isolated from the same individual. The prospect of producing vaccines active against all possible variants of the virus was thought to be an impossibility to achieve, as the constantly changing virus would continue 'slipping away' by changing into new variants.

Another important property of the virus which is a major obstacle to vaccine development is its ability to exist in the form of a latent infection, where its genome is integrated into that of the host cell. In this form the virus is sheltered from the effects of the host's immune system and, like variability, this is a property which helps the virus to evade the immune response of the host. In this case the virus would be largely 'invisible' to the host's immune system.

A further mechanism that the virus exploits to escape the immune response is its propensity to infect sites in the body which are relatively hidden from the immune system, such as the brain. Nervous tissue is somewhat inaccessible to the immune system and it can become a reservoir for persistent infection.

There are a number of theoretical reasons for fearing that a potential HIV vaccine may, in fact, be harmful rather than beneficial. Any protective HIV vaccine would need to consist of gp120 in some form, either as a subunit vaccine or within a multiplying 'carrier' virus such as vaccinia, or as part of a 'killed' virus vaccine. The administration of the gp120 envelope protein or its precursor, gp160 (which is split into gp120 and gp41), especially as a subunit vaccine, may itself be directly immunosuppressive. One of its potentially harmful effects is its ability to fuse cells to each other (to form syncytia) in cell culture. Another potential difficulty with the use of gp120 as an antigen in a vaccine is the fact that its attachment to the CD4 receptor may compete with the physiological function of the antigen-presenting cells attaching to the CD4 receptor of the CD4 lymphocyte to present new antigens to the immune system; gp120 may thus interfere with the normal working of the immune system. An additional fear is the fact that antibodies elicited by gp120 could attach to the surface proteins of the antigen-presenting cells and block their interaction with CD4 antigen. Also, mirror image antibodies directed against the anti-gp120 antibodies could similarly attach to and block CD4 antigen of the CD4 lymphocyte. With either of these mechanisms the immune responses of the host elicited by the vaccine could instead target onto the host itself and cause damage by a disease process called auto-immunity; that is, the immune response acting on the body's own tissues causing pathological effects.

Yet another theoretical danger of any anti-HIV vaccine is the possibility that antibodies produced by such a vaccine may not only be non-neutralizing, but may still be able to attach to the virus and act as a vehicle to transport the virus to monocytes and macrophages which have receptor sites for parts of the antibody molecule (the Fc segment of the antibody molecule). These non-neutralizing antibodies directed against parts of the virus which are not crucial for its replication would thereby facilitate and accelerate the entry of the virus into these cells rather than protect against infection. This process is called antibody enhancement and has been shown to be important in other viral diseases such as dengue and rabies. Its relevance in the pathogenesis of HIV infection, or its importance for future vaccine design, is still uncertain.

To add to all of these theoretical difficulties there are also some problems which are perhaps of relatively lesser importance. The virus is difficult to grow in cell culture and only yields small amounts of viral material in culture. This is in contrast to many presently used vaccines such as poliomyelitis vaccine, which can easily be grown to yield large amounts of virus in cell culture. Thus, unless there is some unforeseen breakthrough in viral culture technology, a future HIV vaccine would probably only be able to be produced by newer recombinant or synthetic technologies. A further reason to exploit the newer technologies for an HIV vaccine in particular is one of safety. The HIV virus suffers from the stigma of belonging to a family of viruses (the Retroviridae) which is associated with malignancy. This association would make the use of the virus itself unsuitable to develop as an attenuated vaccine (even if large scale culture were to become possible), or as a 'killed' or inactivated whole virus vaccine (because the nucleic acid could still be present and the genetic information could hold a theoretical danger of being able to transform cells into malignancy). The Jennerian approach to use one of the SIV strains as a surrogate vaccine, given that they do not produce disease in their natural hosts, would likewise be undesirable. Other animal retroviruses which are more distantly related would have even less potential usefulness. Interestingly enough, the goat retrovirus (called caprine arthritis encephalitis virus) has shown cross-protective activity with HIV, although the relevance of this observation is not clear.

Ethical difficulties

The assessment of efficacy of a potential HIV vaccine in human subjects creates unique ethical problems. The choice of volunteers to take part in such a trial would be highly problematic. Ideally, they would need to be individuals who had not yet been infected, but were at high risk of becoming infected. In developed countries those who could be considered would be homosexual men and intravenous drug abuser groups. However, with the decline in the prevalence of HIV infection in homosexual men and especially amongst those who might be motivated to participate in such a trial, self-motivating behavioural changes may play a greater role in reducing infection than any putative vaccine, and the effect of this would be difficult to distinguish from any possible protective effect of a candidate vaccine. In the case of intravenous drug abusers, where behavioural modifications have not been quite so successful, those individuals likely to be chosen as test subjects, because they remain at high risk of infection, would also be the ones who would be less likely to be able to be traced for follow-up evaluation.

To assess the efficacy of a potential vaccine it would probably be scientifically more advantageous to conduct trials in developing countries where the prevalence is still relatively low but is rising steeply. Such trials would impose particular ethical and moral difficulties. Trials in developing countries could not unreasonably be construed as exploitation of poorer, less developed populations for the purpose of testing of vaccines which would largely benefit the industrialized world (as they would, in the main, be too expensive for the developing world). A commitment to supply, at reasonable cost, the relevant country with a future vaccine would need to be part of the conditions for conducting trials in the developing world.

The evaluation of the efficacy of a candidate vaccine is also beset with problems. The mere act of selecting persons for a vaccine trial would morally and ethically oblige those responsible for the trial to provide adequate education to reduce high-risk behaviour and also to provide condoms to reduce the risk of infection. This, in itself, would substantially lower the risk of HIV infection irrespective of the effect of the vaccine and would markedly bias the significance of any positive findings.

A further ethical dilemma is the fact that individuals who receive vaccine should develop antibodies to HIV, that is they would become HIV positive with all its implications for obtaining insurance, housing loans, employment and immigration. It would, however, usually be possible to distinguish, on Western blot tests, between the antibody response due to a vaccine (which would only have bands for gp160, gp120 or gp41, depending on which vaccine subunits were used) from natural infection (which would also have bands for other viral proteins).

Economic difficulties in producing a vaccine

The manufacture and development of all vaccines have been seriously affected by the huge financial outlays for development and research, the maintenance of the very stringent safety requirements for human vaccines and the enormous costs involved in litigation and insurance for legal costs. There is, in fact, accumulating evidence that the fear of litigation has, itself, significantly retarded the development of anti-HIV vaccines by pharmaceutical companies. It is, therefore, difficult to conceive how any future HIV vaccine would be anything other than expensive, given the enormous cost of research, the resources which have already been spent, the additionally stringent safety requirements which would be needed for the handling and utilization of HIV for deriving a human vaccine and the vulnerability to crippling litigation because of the high public consciousness of AIDS and its implications.

Yet, despite all of these seemingly insuperable obstacles, the gloom of the late 1980s has, to some extent, been lifted by the cautious optimism of the 1990s. This optimism has largely come about from the results of studies in experimental animal models.

Experiment animal models in the development of HIV vaccines

The chimpanzee model of HIV

The chimpanzee is the only animal other than humans which can be infected with HIV and is therefore an extremely valuable animal model of HIV infection. The virus can establish itself in this animal and will elicit an immune response, although there are no symptoms or evidence of immune suppression. The chimpanzee is therefore of great value for studies of the protective immunity of vaccines, as the animal can be immunized with a potential vaccine and the efficacy then examined by challenging with live HIV. However, as no clinical or even laboratory evidence of disease is produced, this animal model cannot be used to study the pathogenic consequences of any challenge infection.

The first vaccine studies on chimpanzees carried out in the second half of the 1980s were almost universally disappointing and added further to the general despondency for the future of an HIV vaccine. A number of studies using a variety of materials to immunize chimpanzees (such as killed whole virus, subunit vaccines, purified peptides and vaccine recombinants) all failed to protect against the challenge virus. Furthermore, little or no immune response could be detected.

In two separate studies carried out in 1989 and 1990 at the Pasteur Institute in France, and at the biotechnology giant, Genentech in the USA, effective immunity was shown to occur if vaccination was given in two steps, a primary vaccination followed by a booster some time later. However, what was also critical to the success of this approach was the requirement that the booster had to consist of peptides comprising what is known as the principal neutralizing determinant (PND). The PND consists essentially of the V3 loop of the gp120 and is so-called because antibodies directed to this sequence of some 30 amino acids will neutralize the infectivity of the virus.

The discovery of the crucial importance of the PND in eliciting neutralizing antibodies, and thus protection, was initially received with profound gloom when it was realized that neutralizing antibodies are highly strain specific and therefore extremely variable from strain to strain. This would therefore impose a virtually impossible obstacle for the design of vaccines. Subsequent findings on the nature of the PND have, however, more recently given cause for a considerable degree of optimism, as some critical neutralizing functions may, in fact, be fairly conserved (that is, not variable between strains). Thus, for example, monoclonal antibodies (antibodies produced by a single clone of antibody-producing B cells and thus exquisitely selective) have been shown to cross-react with the PND from a number of different strains (clades) of HIV.

The V3 loop has now been shown to consist not only of variable sectors but also conserved regions, especially at the crown of the loop. This part of the loop may house the sites of cleavage of the gp120, that is the site where the protein is split open to subsequently expose the fusion protein gp41 and thus allow the virus to penetrate into the cell. This finding therefore means that vaccines could be designed which would elicit antibodies directed against this site, which is crucial for viral replication, and these antibodies should then be able to neutralize the virus. As this site is conserved, variability of the rest of the V3 loop could be bypassed and a single vaccine could possibly be effective for many strains of virus.

Another conserved target for vaccines is the segments of gp120 that are collectively involved in the determination of its folding, or conformation, the specificity of which is similarly crucial for the replication of the virus. This conformational structure governing the ability of the virus to attach to CD4, being also conserved, would allow for a single vaccine to be designed which could be effective against a variety of virus strains.

The chimpanzee model has also been used to demonstrate effective immune protection against challenge by intracellular HIV in the form of HIV-infected cells – the first demonstration of vaccine-induced immunity to cell-associated HIV.

Chimpanzees are, however, now rarely used for vaccine research. They are in very short supply and are enormously expensive to purchase and to rear. As a result experiments have had to be limited to very few animals at a time making it very problematic to evaluate meaningful effects.

The macaque model of AIDS

The rhesus macaque monkey of Asia is not infected with any SIV strain in nature. However, laboratory-reared macaques (Fig. 7.1) can be readily infected with a number of SIV strains, including the original SIVmac strain isolated from laboratory macaques, which produce an AIDS-like disease in these animals. This model of AIDS has proved to be extremely valuable as the clinical elements of the disease are virtually identical to AIDS in humans. If anything, the time course of the disease in the macaque monkey is even more rapid, making it convenient for experimental observations. The

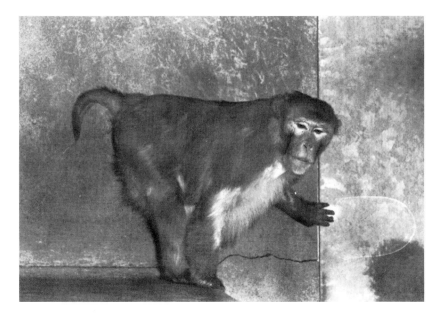

Fig. 7.1 Laboratory-bred rhesus macaque monkey

animals are also more readily obtainable and cheaper to maintain than chimpanzees. Nevertheless there are still doubts as to whether the elements of SIV disease in the macaque are biologically equivalent to AIDS in humans and one would need to be cautious in attempting to extrapolate the findings in the macaque model to those in humans. SIV itself, while it is generally similar to HIV, does differ in some respects; for example, the organization of its genome. Also the V3 loop of SIV does not have a neutralizing determinant as in HIV.

SIV disease in macaques has been a valuable model of human AIDS. It has corroborated the chimpanzee HIV findings, that protection can be achieved against different strains of SIV, thus also demonstrating that the potential obstacle of the variability of the virus could be overcome. The model has also been of particular value in the assessment of the efficacy of protection in the mucosal surfaces. Thus, vaccination by injection has been shown to be successful in preventing the challenge of virus admin- istered via the rectum but not via the vagina. Prevention of vaginal transmission still remains a major obstacle to overcome, as it would be critical to be able to produce effective immunity at all mucosal surfaces if infection is to be prevented by a future vaccine.

The SIV macaque model has also been of value in demonstrating that vaccinated animals may be protected against challenge virus administered in the form of infected cells, as with HIV and the chimpanzee model. Thus, there is further corroboration that another potential hurdle, that of intracellular virus being sheltered from the immune response, could potentially also be overcome.

One of the more recent exciting developments in vaccine research has been the development of a hybrid virus which consists of the envelope of HIV virus together with the remaining component of the SIV virus; this hybrid is called the 'SHIV' virus. It infects and causes disease in macaque monkeys as does SIV, but SHIV elicits a protective immune response to HIV because of the HIV envelope component and is thus particularly useful in studying the immune protection afforded by putative vaccines.

These animal experiments have been able to establish the feasibility of an HIV vaccine by demonstrating that a number of the daunting theoretical obstacles to vaccine development, such as virus variability, intracellular location and even, to some extent, immune protection against the establishment of latent infection, can be overcome in practice. Nevertheless, one would need to be very cautious in not extrapolating too closely from animal model studies.

Experimental HIV vaccines

As mentioned above, because of safety concerns about retroviruses, there has been relatively little effort put into developing a live attenuated HIV vaccine or to utilizing other animal retroviruses for the development of a human vaccine on the Jennerian principle. For similar reasons there has also been a reluctance to develop killed or inactivated HIV vaccines. The majority of HIV vaccine developments have therefore concentrated on subunit vaccines, investigating various antigens of the virus, or recombinant live viruses consisting of vectors (carriers) of genes coding for important antigens of HIV, as well as DNA vaccines.

Subunit vaccines

Most HIV vaccine trials have involved subunit vaccines consisting of the surface glycoproteins of HIV – the gp160 or gp140 or a combination of both. These antigens contain the neutralizing domains and, being the outermost antigens of the virus, they would be the proteins most likely to elicit protective immune responses. However, because they are also the most variable of the antigens, vaccines that are based on these proteins would be the ones that would be the most strain specific in their immune responses.

Other parts of the virus that have been investigated are the gp41 glyco-protein and, more recently, the internal proteins of the virus such as the *gag* protein which shows the least variation between strains.

Recombinant vaccines

A number of live virus and even bacterial vectors have been examined as possible carriers of protective antigens of HIV. The vaccinia virus, which was used as a vaccine against smallpox and which successfully eradicated smallpox from the planet, is an attractive option. The virus is very large (by viral standards) and it is therefore comparatively easy to genetically recombine foreign genes into the genome of the virus such as those from HIV. The resultant vaccine replicates well and produces a strong immune response in the host, both antibody as well as cell-mediated immune responses. The protection is generally relatively broad and not narrowly strain specific as in the case of the subunit vaccines alone. Another important advantage of vaccinia is that it is relatively easy to administer – the vaccine is scratched into the skin – as was demonstrated so successfully in the smallpox eradication campaign by relatively untrained personnel. Unfortunately the one drawback of vaccinia itself is that it is not entirely innocuous and some unpleasant side-effects may occur, and on occasion these side-effects may be serious. A related strain of virus, the canarypox virus, is being viewed as an attractive alternative to vaccinia, as it has the same virological properties as vaccinia with respect to genetic recombination, but is quite harmless to humans.

The prime-boost regimen of vaccination has been shown in a number of experiments in macaques challenged with the SHIV hybrid virus to be highly effective in inducing protective immunity. For priming the immune system, a recombinant canarypox vaccine containing gp160/120 is used, followed a little while later with a booster to the immune system consisting of the purified gp160/120 subunit vaccine. Neutralizing antibodies as well as cytotoxic lymphocytes are induced.

DNA vaccines

Naked DNA HIV vaccines have been investigated in experimental animal models. These vaccines can be produced relatively inexpensively in large amounts and when injected into the muscle or skin elicit strong antibody and cell-mediated immune responses to challenge SHIV. A strong neutralizing antibody response and cytotoxic T lymphocyte response is induced. However, technical obstacles need to be overcome with respect to difficulties in administration and specifically the need for very large amounts of DNA to be injected.

Human trials of potential HIV vaccines

Human resistance to HIV infection

There has been intense interest in a number of observed cases of apparent resistance to HIV infection. These individuals have been rigorously studied as they could provide very important information regarding natural immunity to the virus which would be of great value in the development of an effective human vaccine. Examples of these persons include infants born to HIV-infected mothers who do not themselves become infected (about a third of infants born to HIV-positive mothers become infected). There are also cases of infants who have been proven to have been infected after birth but then subsequently overcome the infection and clear the virus from their bodies. Presumably there are also adults who are able to overcome HIV infection, although this has not yet been clearly documented because most HIV infections are asymptomatic and therefore adults who have lost the infection would generally not be aware that they had previously been infected. Perhaps the most directly visible example of apparent resistance are the sexually promiscuous persons who continue to indulge in frequent high-risk practices but remain HIV negative. A number of groups of these individuals have been closely researched; for example, prostitutes in Kenya and Guinea Bissau, and homosexual men in San Francisco. Lastly there are a number of examples of discordant couples in stable relationships where one partner is HIV positive and the other sexual partner remains negative despite a continuing sexual relationship.

Some, but not all, of these individuals have mutations in the CCR-5 co-receptor for HIV (discussed in Chapters 3 and 4) which could be an explanation for their resistance to HIV infection. In many resistant persons a strong cytotoxic T lymphocyte (CTL) immune response to HIV can be demonstrated in spite of the absence of antibodies. This would suggest that cell-mediated immunity is important in resisting HIV infection and a strong CTL response would need to be a requirement for an effective vaccine in addition to the production of neutralizing antibodies.

Human vaccine trials

Human trials of potential HIV vaccines often receive very wide publicity in the press and nearly always mislead the public into a belief that these trials indicate the imminence of a vaccine 'breakthrough'. There are a number of phase I and phase II vaccine trials being conducted in humans in various centres in the USA and Europe. The terms phase I, phase II and phase III are used for vaccine trials in a similar way to drug trials (see

Chapter 6). Phase I trials assess the safety of a candidate vaccine and evaluate its side-effects in humans. Phase II trials assess the immunogenicity
(the ability and the efficacy in eliciting an immune response) and phase III
the protective efficacy by observing the rate of infection in vaccinated
subjects as compared to that in control non-infected subjects.

Preliminary results of the phase I and II studies have, to date, been highly
encouraging. A number of candidate vaccines have been evaluated, including subunit vaccines and recombinant vaccinia vaccines.

The ethical and related difficulties in carrying out phase III trials in
human populations have been discussed previously. Nevertheless the WHO,
in spite of these difficulties as well as the incompleteness of animal studies and human phase I and phase II studies, planned for the conducting of
efficacy trials in the mid-1990s because of the very pressing urgency to at
least make a start with evaluating the effectiveness of potential vaccines.
Four developing countries were selected for large scale vaccine trials –
Brazil, Rwanda, Thailand and Uganda, as well as the USA. These phase
III trials were suspended, but are now scheduled to recommence towards
the end of 1998 or early 1999.

Post-infection vaccination

The concept of immunizing individuals who have already been infected was
first mooted in 1987 by Jonas Salk, the inventor of the poliomyelitis vaccine, to delay or even prevent the onset of AIDS disease. An increasing
number of HIV-infected persons have been observed who remain asymptomatic for over 10 to 20 years with reasonably preserved immune function.
These long-term non-progressors have vigorous cell-mediated immune
responses (Th1 responses – see Chapter 3) which prevent the disease process
progressing to AIDS. Post-infection vaccination attempts to mimic this natural resistance by stimulating the cellular immune system. In preliminary
studies in symptomatically infected individuals, some relief of symptoms
followed the injection of killed whole virus vaccines, possibly due to the
stimulation of the immune system. Recently, immunization of asymptomatically infected individuals with a gp160 subunit vaccine produced gratifyingly high levels of specific antibodies. The status and possible benefits
of post-infection vaccination, however, still need to be determined.

The future of HIV vaccines

After a period of despondency due to theoretical obstacles which appeared
to be insurmountable, as well as failed animal experiments, the outlook

for vaccines now appears to be considerably brighter. The difficulties of virus variability, intracellular shelter and, to some extent, latency can apparently be addressed, although not as yet overcome. Animal experiments have now demonstrated some considerable success and even preliminary phase I and phase II human studies have been encouraging. Phase III efficacy trials are in the planning stage and should commence in the near future.

Nevertheless, there still remain major obstacles and considerable gaps in our knowledge. The relevance of the variable regions of the PND, the protective ability of antibodies directed to conserved regions of PND and the conformational antigens involved in CD4 binding, the potential harmful effects of gp120 and auto-immunity, as well as a number of other issues still remain to be elucidated both in the laboratory and in experimental animals. The major ethical issues discussed above are also still unresolved and the enormous financial obstacles still need to be addressed.

There is however, at present, a guarded optimism that a utilizable vaccine could well be available in the not-too-distant future. On May 18, 1997, United States President, Bill Clinton, called for a commitment to develop an HIV vaccine 'within the next decade'. The attainment of this goal would be an even more valuable achievement than the fulfilment of President Kennedy's pledge three decades previously of putting a man on the moon.

8

The ethics of AIDS

The ethics of human behaviour are, in a broad sense, governed by two opposing needs. On the one hand there are the fundamental human civil rights of the individual for freedom and a desire for an unfettered and unrestricted existence. On the other hand lie the needs of the community for regulations and laws to restrain those individual activities which may be to the detriment of the common good. In essence, it is the resolution of these two opposing necessities that governs the ethical framework for regulating human behaviour – a framework which exhibits vast differences in different populations with varying cultures, socio-political systems, economic resources and religious beliefs.

Public health legislation for communicable diseases

Human responses to contagious diseases

Contagious diseases have, since antiquity, exerted a profound effect on community behaviour, mainly in the direction of panic and mass flight from epidemics. Right up to the twentieth century, scenes of irrational hysteria have been witnessed; for example, in the USA during the poliomyelitis epidemic of the 1930s and 1940s where children were stampeded, and even forcibly removed from affected cities and, in some instances, armed vigilante groups 'protected' unaffected cities.

The terror associated with these contagions also brought out all that was vile and debased in humankind, and gave rise to some of the most horrific acts of torture and butchery in human history. Since ancient times, scapegoats have been sought to exculpate the community from responsibility for epidemics. In the plague which swept Europe in the fourteenth century, the Jews were accused of poisoning the wells, and in the nineteenth and twentieth centuries it was the newly arrived Italian immigrants who were blamed for the introduction of poliomyelitis into America. Together with this fear, superstition and ignorance came the discrimination, victimization and persecution so typical of human behaviour under stress. These elements of fear, scapegoating and victimization are no less relevant to the modern-day plague of AIDS.

The development of public health laws

Infectious or communicable diseases are a phenomenon of humankind, where the rights of the individual may well clash quite starkly with the needs of the community. Diseases that have the potential to be transmitted to other individuals no longer fall within the personal and private interests of the individual alone. The personal civil liberties would now have to be limited and restricted for the benefit or protection of society in no less a way than traffic regulations, rules of public decency or any of the myriad of society's civil and criminal laws.

Many of the public health laws governing the control of infectious diseases were framed towards the end of the nineteenth and early twentieth centuries. Further statutes, regulations and various court decisions have contributed to produce the measures that were taken to limit the spread of communicable diseases. Public health administrators were thus provided with powers for compulsory testing or routine screening for designated infectious diseases, and mandatory reporting of notifiable conditions to authorities with appropriate penalties for failing to comply. Statutory provisions do often directly infringe on civil liberties. For example, infected individuals may, where necessary, be confined or isolated and even those suspected to be infected may be quarantined. Public health laws have also provided officials with mandates to inspect food establishments, crèches and nursing homes and also powers to shut these institutions down if regulations are not adequately complied with. Individuals who are chronically infected with salmonella are forbidden to work as food handlers until such time as an inspector would designate them as being free from infection. Until recent times there has, in general, been little opposition or controversy with the majority of public health legislation. Few would contest the morality of depriving an individual of his or her rights by confining or quarantining a person who is infected with a viral haemorrhagic fever or plague.

These public health enactments have, in the main, been framed to address the control of infectious diseases. Some specific regulations have been applied to sexually transmitted diseases, as for example the provision for contact tracing, that is, tracing of sexual contacts of infected persons by public health officials for the purposes of counselling and, if necessary, treatment.

Largely due to the advances in therapy and vaccination and the consequent falling away of the need for many of these measures, as well as the changing concepts of civil liberties and rights, the enforcement of many public health provisions has been considerably relaxed. There was, at any rate, little controversy in response to most of the restrictions that applied to communicable diseases, because the contagiousness was readily apparent and also most conditions were of a temporary nature and often of quite a short duration so that restrictions were usually viewed as not much more than an inconvenience.

Public health laws and AIDS

With the rapid advances of medical science and its spectacular successes in controlling infectious diseases by drugs and vaccines, the issues of public health intrusions into human rights and civil liberties has largely receded. The advent of the AIDS epidemic has, however, dramatically re-focused attention with a renewed intensity onto the age-old conflicts between the rights of protection of the health of the public and the rights of the individual. AIDS resembles the plague of the Middle Ages in that it is also incurable, lethal and has the potential to cause the same kind of mass death and destruction. It also resembles the ancient plagues in causing people and groups to be blamed, victimized and discriminated against.

Thus, while in more modern times public health measures applied to control communicable diseases met with relatively little opposition or controversy, these same measures applied to AIDS have radically different implications for two reasons – the characteristics of the disease and the characteristics of individuals who are predominantly infected. These characteristics of AIDS, which distinguish it from other infectious diseases, are: firstly, that it is lethal and incurable; secondly, that it is a life-long infection with life-long infectiousness; and thirdly, that infectivity is so low that the risk of infection can voluntarily be virtually eliminated by the behaviours and habits of the individual. Because AIDS is an incurable and lethal infectious disease, it instils fear and panic, as did the plagues of ancient times, and provokes irrational behaviour and illogical suggestions for solutions. Because the infection and the infectivity are of life-long duration, it makes certain public health options, such as isolation or quarantining, unworkable. Because the transmissibility of the virus is so low, it implies that the majority of infected individuals have acquired infection by their own free-will choice and therefore would have only themselves to blame. It aggravates the victimization of infected individuals and those perceived by society to be at risk of infection, who are then blamed for the spread of the disease and for placing the 'rest' of society at risk of being 'involuntarily' infected, for example by blood transfusion.

Therefore, the characteristics of the individuals who are predominantly affected by AIDS clearly form a dominant feature in differentiating it from other infectious diseases. The psycho-social segregating of those who choose to put themselves at risk of infection and those who can comfort themselves that AIDS is a problem of those individuals who deserve it is a pervasive feeling in much of the developed world, where the great majority of infections are still found in homosexual men, intravenous drug abusers and their sexual consorts. That the major spread of infection into the heterosexual population of the developed world, which was widely predicted to occur, has still not really materialized to any great extent (despite the fact that it remains the most rapidly growing infected group in the developed world) has only served to strengthen the isolation of the 'at risk' groups. In many developed countries, such as the USA, the disease has, in more recent times, expanded most rapidly into the disadvantaged inner city populations and especially amongst non-white people. Thus, groups categorized as 'Black' and 'Hispanic' constituted some 61% of all AIDS cases reported in the USA in 1996, while they comprised only 20% of the country's total population. Sub-Saharan Africa, with less than 10% of the planet's population, is estimated to house over 60% of the world's HIV infections. Not surprisingly, therefore, racism has now joined the other more traditional AIDS discriminations and victimizations and has spawned bumper stickers such as 'Thank God for AIDS'.

All these specific and peculiar features of AIDS have had a marked influence on the modification of the traditional public health measures that are used to control infectious diseases. AIDS has thus become an exception to the general rules of infectious diseases and has created for itself a separate and unique ethical framework.

The ethics of AIDS, which defines the public response and the code of behaviour to the disease and those that it affects, are themselves largely governed by the politics of AIDS which, in turn, reflect the perceptions, the needs and the wishes of the population. The politics of AIDS, in turn, manifest themselves in the formal laws and regulations that are enacted at a national or regional level, the rules laid down at a local or institutional level, and also the codes of behaviour at an individual level.

In the final analysis, the ethics, politics and legislation of AIDS have, in general, been the result of the merging of the traditions of public health infectious disease control and a respect for the societal values of civil liberties, the rights of individuals to protection from discrimination and also the right to privacy. As the ethics of human behaviour, in general, have varied vastly between countries, so too are there immense differences in the ethical responses to the AIDS epidemic. For example, at the one extreme the notorious Cuban approach to AIDS control consists of mandatory screening, initially of groups categorized as 'high risk', but ultimately the entire population. All individuals found to be HIV infected are then quarantined, presumably for life, in a specially designated sanatorium in the outskirts of Havana. In contrast, in The Netherlands and Denmark, the respect for privacy has extended, for example, to forbidding doctors from disclosing an HIV result even if that individual refuses to do so himself and thereby endangers a sexual partner; also decisions were made not to close down or to even regulate the notorious bathhouses, such places being closed in the USA because they were used for promiscuous, anonymous sexual contacts.

Individual and group viewpoints on AIDS control vary even more widely than national policies and largely reflect political orientations and, to some extent, religious convictions. The rightwing of political opinion in most western countries nearly always advocates AIDS being subject to the same public health controls as other sexually transmitted and infectious diseases. That AIDS is a lethal and incurable disease which is progressively spreading is seen as an even more urgent reason for the need to protect the public at all costs rather than to grant AIDS extraordinary privileges. The public health establishment is frequently accused by this body of opinion of capitulating to the pressures and demands of vocal and articulate pressure groups in the gay community.

The liberal traditions in countries of the world argue, on the other hand, that coercive public health measures have time and again proved counterproductive not only with HIV but also with syphilis and other sexually transmitted diseases and infectious diseases. These measures cannot be enforced without loss of privacy and the ripple effects, which often lead to the destruction of people's lives and those of their families. This can only widen the gulf of suspicion and distrust of the state and its agencies, including the medical profession, and thus drive the disease even further from being accessible to any control measures.

The effect of religious traditions does itself vary amongst different beliefs. In general, theologians espouse a philosophy of caring, compassion and sensitivity to those who are infected, but a condemnation of the activities which are characteristically associated with the transmission of the virus. Religions generally condemn discrimination and nearly always oppose victimization. The influence of religion on legislation associated with AIDS has been strongest in countries where religion dominates the culture of the society, such as many Islamic countries where, for example, educational programmes would be profoundly affected, or some Catholic countries where condom distribution and advertising would be prohibited.

Ethico-legal approaches to balancing community rights and individual rights

Statutory notification

The mandatory reporting of diseases of public health importance has long been held to be a very important component of health monitoring and surveillance. The lists of notifiable conditions do vary somewhat from country to country, but generally include the formidable epidemic diseases such as the viral haemorrhagic fevers and plague, the vaccine-preventable diseases where monitoring of disease would be a marker of the success of vaccination programmes such as those for poliomyelitis and measles, and even some non-infectious diseases, such as insecticide poisoning, where rapid public health responses can prevent further disease from occurring.

There is little controversy about the need for health authorities to have information on the extent of AIDS and the spread and behaviour of the epidemic. AIDS has been a reportable disease, with few objections, in every state of the USA since 1983. Reporting of AIDS is also mandatory in the majority of developed countries of the world, the major exception being the United Kingdom.

The reporting of AIDS cases by name to health authorities has not been particularly vigorously opposed as it is highly unlikely that a patient with AIDS coming for treatment to a hospital will anyway be able to maintain anonymity. However, the mandatory reporting of individuals with asymptomatic HIV infection has been strongly resisted by advocates for human rights. In a number of states in the USA, Australia, some provinces of Canada and some European, Asian and Central American countries, there are statutory provisions for the reporting of HIV positivity. In some countries, for example Sweden, HIV reporting is carried out by means of an anonymous coding system. Most countries that do not have statutory notification provisions acquire data on AIDS cases and numbers of HIV-infected individuals through voluntary reporting on an anonymous basis by doctors and laboratories. Whether voluntary reporting is any less accurate than statutory notification remains to be established.

Antibody screening

Mass screening for HIV antibodies is carried out under many guises. Some screening programmes exist for the benefit of the individual, for example antenatal screening or newborn screening. In other cases, the screening is for the benefit of a direct contact, such as pre-marital screening, or the testing of sex offenders. Screening is also carried out for the benefit of society as a whole, as in the case of epidemiological screening to obtain information, or screening of migrants for the 'protection' of the population, the screening of prostitutes to protect clients and screening programmes in prisons to protect fellow inmates. Economic motives form the basis of pre-employment screening and insurance screening.

Of all these screening programmes, those involving the routine testing of pregnant mothers is probably one of the least controversial, provided it is carried out with her consent after the woman has been counselled and adequately informed of the implications of the test and the possibilities of a positive result. Ethically, antenatal screening would be relatively readily justifiable on the grounds that the management of the pregnancy (including decisions to terminate pregnancy) would be directly affected by knowledge of the HIV status. On ethical grounds, the routine screening of newborn babies is somewhat more problematical even though knowledge that an infant is infected could directly affect its clinical management, for example with early prophylaxis against *Pneumocystis carinii* pneumonia. The ethical difficulties are largely due to the technical shortcomings of presently available routine testing which, in effect, test for infection in the mother. Maternal antibodies cannot be distinguished from those made by the infant, should it be infected, until after 15 months *post-partum* when the mother's antibodies would have disappeared (as discussed in Chapter 5). If tests for viral infection in infants alone were to become routinely available, ethical objections to routine neonatal screening would be greatly reduced.

Testing of sex offenders for HIV infection is routinely carried out in most countries. It is, of course, generally accepted to be unethical to test an alleged assailant without their agreement, although mandatory testing is often sanctioned when such a case comes to court.

Ethical considerations regarding epidemiological screening will be discussed in Chapter 9. The ethics of HIV screening and the providing of an HIV result as a condition of entry into a country, on a temporary or permanent basis, has always been fraught with controversy and has provoked violent opposition. In the USA, legislation requiring an HIV-negative test result for immigration purposes has become a major issue of discontent among both gay rights protagonists and civil libertarians, and was also responsible for the moving of the venue for the VIIIth International Congress on AIDS in 1992, at a late hour, from Boston to Amsterdam. In South Africa, mandatory screening of migrants was instituted by the pre-1994 regime to protect the country from the feared southward migration of HIV infection, by attempting to create a kind of 'cordon sanitaire'. The ineffectiveness of such a barrier was soon realized and the regulation was subsequently repealed. Not only are there strong moral objections to the practice of screening of migrants, but there is little scientific logic to support it, as the small numbers of incoming infected individuals would have no meaningful epidemiological effect on the HIV status of the host country. Screening of sex workers (prostitutes) is clearly an important component of their regular medical care. One of the major motivations for legalizing prostitution is to enable regular health monitoring to be instituted. HIV screening of prisoners is routinely carried out in most prisons with or without informed consent. Coercive testing in these settings remains controversial even though it is almost universally practised. However, even more problematic is the subsequent handling of HIV-positive prisoners.

Screening for HIV infection has become the universal practice of insurance companies throughout the world for policies exceeding a moderate value. In theory, there should be few grounds for objecting to the testing for a chronic illness which could quite likely produce disability and a reduced life span, any more than the routine testing for similar chronic conditions such as diabetes or hypertension. There has, however, been some quite robust resistance to HIV screening for insurance policies by civil rights advocates. However, routine pre-employment screening for HIV has provoked very much stronger objections. Pre-employment screening is usually mooted for on one of three grounds. Firstly, as an important part of a legitimate routine medical examination to assess the health status of a prospective employee and to safeguard the company's interests, such as its medical benefits, disability and pension funds. Secondly, to protect against health-related deterioration of job performance, especially in those jobs requiring a high degree of mental alertness which could be affected by impairments in neurophysiological functioning, even in asymptomatically infected individuals (see Chapter 1). For this reason the HIV status could be held to be particularly crucial in applications for jobs involving heavy machinery or where public safety could be endangered, such as those of airline pilots and bus drivers. The third reason given to justify pre-employment screening is to 'protect' workers from acquiring infection in the workplace; for example, should the nature of the work be such that there may be a significant risk of injury with the potential of exposing fellow workers to infected blood.

Routine pre-employment screening has been rejected by a wide spectrum of opinion. Irrespective of assurances to the contrary, confidentiality cannot be guaranteed and the recording of an HIV-positive test result in an employee's staff record undoubtedly constitutes a flagrant violation of that person's rights to privacy, quite different from that of other medical conditions which may be placed on record but do not carry the same stigma and social consequences as HIV infection. None of these three reasons provides sufficient justification for pre-employment HIV screening. Screening cannot furnish adequate assurance against infection, which could occur at any time after testing, and ongoing testing would be impractical. Safeguards could be introduced into medical aid and disability funds such as, for example, placing a limit on the payments for AIDS-related conditions. Individuals in high-risk occupations involving public safety should have regular neurophysiological testing independent of HIV infection. There is no scientific basis for HIV testing to protect workers from transmission of HIV in the workplace, as there is virtually no risk of infection in any work-related interpersonal contact, even, for example, accidental contact with blood as a result of injuries with blood spills, especially if facilities for universal blood precautions are available where there is a risk of work-related injuries.

Legislated restrictions on individuals

There is a common feeling amongst those of reactionary political persuasion that the only way of curtailing the epidemic would be to use the same measures that are used with other infectious diseases and sexually transmitted diseases, into both of which categories AIDS unquestionably falls. Bizarre measures such as the routine quarantining of infected patients into special sanatoria is only practised in Cuba but is nevertheless something which many would propose as a solution to stopping the transmission of the virus. Quarantining in the HIV context implies life-long incarceration or restraint. Clearly this course of action would constitute a profound affront to any reasonable system of human values. It would reflect a brutal public response to an individual who would have his or her liberty forcibly removed from them, not because he or she had committed any offence but because of an infection; not because of what they had done but what they may do in the future. Not surprisingly, no state authority anywhere in the world, other than Cuba, has pursued any such policy.

Legalized restrains have, however, been enforced in certain special circumstances, such as where an infected person either deliberately seeks to infect others, for example for revenge, or where they are mentally disturbed, or are unwilling or feel unable to stop prostitution or simply refuse to adopt precautions to protect others and continue with their high-risk activities. Some of these attempts at restraining the activities of high-risk, recalcitrant individuals have received considerable publicity. For example, the use of an electronic device that a number of infected prostitutes have been forced to wear in parts of the USA, which signals an alarm to the police should they move more than a pre-determined distance away from a phone. In other instances various forms of 'house arrest' have been attempted where recalcitrant individuals have been legally confined to a house or neighbourhood. Not unexpectedly, bizarre suggestions have also been forthcoming such as castration or mutilation for infected men who are habitual sex offenders.

AIDS ethical issues in medical practice

Among the most intractable and divisive of the ethical dilemmas in the field of AIDS are those which concern the relationship between the doctor and other health care workers and the HIV-infected patient. Some of these issues have rocked the very foundations of the medical profession like no other single disease before it, and have opened up huge chasms between different factions within the profession and also between the profession and the public.

Broadly speaking there are two main ethical issues which affect the relationship between the disease of AIDS and the health care professions. Firstly, the conflict between the rights of the doctor and related health care workers to protection from HIV infection *versus* the rights of the infected patient to privacy and a freedom from fear of discrimination. (Related to this is the right of the patient to be protected from an infected doctor.) Secondly, the conflict between the professional obligation of the doctor to respect patient confidentiality as against his or her moral responsibility to breach that confidentiality when necessary to prevent the transmission of a lethal infection.

The right of the doctor to protection from HIV infection

There are very few members of the health care professions who would deny that their vocation does not entail a certain degree of personal risk. These risks come in a number of forms. For example, exposure to radiation is a hazard which radiotherapists, radiologists and radiographers accept as an intrinsic component of their work. The danger of contracting an infectious disease is one to which all health care workers have always been exposed to a lesser or greater extent depending on the nature of their particular speciality. Certainly, in ancient times, great risks were taken by doctors attending to the sick and the dying during the formidable plagues of earlier times, and indeed many were infected and succumbed. Right up until the advent of the antibiotic era, the practice of medicine entailed a significant hazard due to the transmission of infections to doctors for which no cure was available. The rapid development of highly effective antibiotics from the second half of the twentieth century coupled with the triumph of vaccines over many of the serious epidemic infectious diseases of the past gave doctors a feeling of invincibility against these erstwhile hazards. It is true that some hazards still remained. Hepatitis B virus infection, for example, was in 1990 still responsible for 6500 to 9000 infections per year in health care workers, of whom 150 died; yet less than 50% of doctors availed themselves of the effective and safe vaccine against this infection. Occasionally doctors also contract severe infections from their patients, meningococcal infections, tuberculosis, hepatitis C and typhoid fever. However, these relatively uncommon infections did little to dent the cosy, reassuring feelings that doctors were very unlikely to contract a serious infection from a patient and, at any rate, modern medicine could always be relied on to take care of the problem. The AIDS epidemic dramatically changed these perceptions. The medical profession was once again thrown back to the era of vulnerability to infectious diseases for which it had no weapons of combat. The vulnerability and helplessness against an incurable infectious disease was a risk which doctors were now not willing to take so glibly. The attempts to educate doctors that the risks were very small, many orders of magnitude smaller than those of hepatitis B, and that the organism is delicate and only transmissible with great difficulty have generally failed to really provide much reassurance. The spectre of contracting HIV infection in the course of one's work remains so overwhelming in its implications for a young doctor and his or her family that reassurances from research scientists have usually been curtly dismissed. As a result a rift in the medical profession has developed between those at the 'coalface' of risk, the surgeons and obstetricians who regularly and frequently sustain needle-stick injuries during operating procedures or splashes of blood in emergency room crises, and, on the other hand, the medical ethicists and the academic fraternity, often portrayed as opining from their comfortable and protected vantage points. Within the medical profession, there are those who advocate routine screening of all patients admitted to hospitals, with or without their consent, and labelling all positive patients to alert health care workers to take especial care in handling them. This would also allow for surgical procedures to be appropriately modified, for example avoiding the use of needles for suturing and instead using staples for closing incision wounds, or having more senior and experienced surgeons operating on these infected patients, who would be placed at the end of an operating list. In certain circumstances surgery would be avoided altogether; for example, not installing orthopaedic prostheses in HIV-infected patients because they are said to be more likely to be accompanied by secondary infection due to suppression of the immune system. This identifying of infected patients and their being singled out for especially careful handling is held to be the only realistic way of preventing the type of accidents which may lead to transmission of infection, as it is impossible to treat all patients in a hospital as if they were positive and to sustain a heightened level of vigilance. The potential loss of privacy and risk of possible consequences of divulging an HIV result would be but a small price to pay for the protection which health care workers are entitled to. The benefits of the HIV test to the patient (see Chapter 5) are an additional motivation for routine testing.

The opposing medical viewpoint objects strongly to this abrogation of the fundamental medical ethical right to privacy and the inevitable stigmatization which would follow the labelling or 'branding' of a patient as being HIV positive, irrespective of what measures may be offered to keep the diagnosis confidential. Also, despite measures to the contrary, the fear of becoming infected from a patient would undoubtedly result in such patients receiving a lower standard of medical care than non-infected patients. Furthermore, reliance on testing has its own dangers if infected patients fail to be detected during screening procedures, either because of the 'window period', that is before antibodies have developed, or because of a falsely negative test result. The false sense of security and relaxation of precautionary measures could increase the risk of accidental transmission of infection. The HIV test should only be recommended when there are specific clinical indications for it, but not for the sole purpose of protecting medical staff. Also, tests should only be carried out when the patient has given voluntary consent after all the implications of a positive result have been fully explained. Health care workers should be protected by the rigorous practising of what are called universal blood precautions. These are a set of procedures devised by the Centers for Disease Control (CDC) in the USA to minimize the risk of accidents with penetrating injuries. All patients admitted to hospital should be regarded as being potentially infectious, and universal blood precautions should always be practised. The labelling of patients to identify them as being HIV positive is strongly opposed and is regarded as a flagrant violation of medical ethics and an unnecessary deprivation of the patient's rights, with no real scientific evidence that the risk to health care workers is really lowered.

No professional or official body has approved of routine screening of all patients admitted to hospitals although in practice it is regularly carried out all over the world. In many hospitals warning notices are displayed advising patients that routine screening is part of hospital policy and a condition of admission. Some bodies, such as the British Medical Association and the Royal College of Surgeons of Scotland, have sanctioned the testing of the blood of a patient without necessarily obtaining consent in the extraordinary circumstance where a needle-stick or similar injury has been sustained by a health care worker and there is a need to determine the HIV status of the source patient.

The rights of the patient to be protected from an HIV-infected health care worker

The rights of a patient to be informed of the HIV status of his or her medical attendant was rarely considered before the well publicized case of the Florida dentist, first reported in July 1990. In this incident a homosexual male dentist was demonstrated to have transmitted the infection to six of his patients, and possibly a further one. However, even after intensive investigations, the routes of transmission have still not been established. This case remains the only documented instance of transmission of infection from a health care worker to a patient. A number of carefully executed studies to investigate patients of infected surgeons involving some 1955 patients as well as a number of more informal studies have universally failed to demonstrate any incidents of infection having been transmitted to any of these patients. The actual risk to a patient of contracting HIV from the blood of an infected health care worker during an invasive surgical procedure is difficult to calculate, given that the Florida dentist was the only such incident. In addition to the risk of transmission of HIV, a further problem of the infected health care worker is that of the possibility of their compromised mental competence, given the possibility that subtle neurophysiological damage could occur in HIV infection (although the WHO has taken a stand that there is no established evidence of this – see Chapter 1). In reality, the chances of a successful outcome of operation may often be greater with a skilful HIV-infected surgeon than a less skilful non-infected surgeon. A number of medical associations, such as the American Medical Association and the British Medical Association, have recommended that infected doctors should not work in specialities which may involve any surgical procedures because of the minute risk of transmission of infection to patients. However, routine testing of health care workers is not warranted, nor is the patient entitled to demand the knowledge of the HIV status of the medical attendant.

Ethical issues of confidentiality

Enshrined in the Hippocratic oath is the solemn undertaking of doctors to preserve the confidentiality of their patients. Until the AIDS era this resolve not to divulge confidential information was seldom tested outside of the law courts where doctors would be compelled, in many countries, to breach confidentiality to serve the ends of justice. In some countries, such as The Netherlands and Denmark, the right of the patient to confidentiality remains absolute irrespective of circumstances. However, in most parts of the world, the doctor may be permitted to breach the confidentiality of their patient to divulge HIV status to a spouse or sexual partner, should the patient refuse to do so. Indeed, in a number of legal systems, the failure to divulge information to a threatened sexual partner could be construed in itself as a misdemeanour. A similar obligation would also exist with other at-risk partners; for example, needle-sharing partners of intravenous drug abusers.

However, a more difficult ethical dilemma confronting the doctor is whether there is an obligation to divulge the HIV status of a patient who is referred to a fellow health care worker. A number of court decisions have been handed down which generally have found in favour of a health care worker having the right, if not the obligation, to warn a colleague of a patient's HIV status.

An ethical difficulty even less clearly defined involves the rights of the doctor to conceal a diagnosis of AIDS or HIV infection on a death certificate, insurance application or related document. It is well known that death certificates are a notoriously inaccurate source of data for AIDS-related mortality because the cause of death in AIDS patients is seldom given as AIDS, but is usually camouflaged as one of the opportunistic infections. However, a more contentious difficulty for the doctor arises when he or she needs to sign an insurance policy or similar document where the wording may compel him or her either to make a false statement, or else breach the confidentiality of their patient's HIV status.

The ethics of the cost of AIDS

The high costs of the treatment of AIDS as well as AIDS research have created their own ethical questions. The life-time cost of treating an AIDS patient in a developed country (USA) in 1992–1993 was estimated to be of the order of $70000, 49% of which was for drugs and 32% for hospitalization. Inevitably conflicts will arise, as they have done with other expensive and restricted treatments, such as renal dialysis, where therapeutic programmes may well compete with each other for limited resources. Inadequate expenditure by health care authorities for AIDS treatment and AIDS research has been an issue in the forefront of protests by activist groups. Nevertheless, calculations published as far back as 1989 have shown that the estimated federal spending in the USA on AIDS and HIV was $1.31 billion while the infection was responsible for 34 388 deaths, compared to $1.01 billion which was spent on heart disease which caused 777 626 deaths and cancer, where $1.54 billion was spent and the disease caused 494 422 deaths.

The ethical dilemmas of the distribution of meagre health resources in the developing world, which is already wracked by other diseases, malnutrition and woefully inadequate social facilities, are even more formidable. There is undoubtedly a far greater priority for preventive health programmes, including programmes for AIDS, as well as immunization, nutrition and other primary health care programmes, as compared to treatment costs for AIDS.

Perhaps the most fundamental ethical challenge of all is that of the inequality and maldistribution of health care resources between the developed world and the developing world, as exemplified in particular by their relative expenditures on AIDS. Thus, about 92% of all expenditure on AIDS, worldwide, takes place in the developed world, even though 80% of all new cases of AIDS occur in the Third World. The average costs of treatment for an AIDS patient in the developed world is $32 000, as compared to $400 or less in Africa.

The religious dimensions of AIDS

More than any other disease in modern history, AIDS has interacted in a profound way with religious doctrine and practice. The pastoral duties of the clergy have frequently brought them into close interpersonal contact with sick and dying AIDS patients, the majority of whom would have acquired their infections through activities which are diametrically opposed to the teachings of the world's major religions. Frequently gay AIDS patients yearn to return to religion but are alienated by the fear of its stern dictates against homosexuality. Religion may well become a factor which exacerbates the pain of the disease.

Another difficulty between religion and AIDS is the conflict around the measures that are taken to control the epidemic. Explicit education which may be regarded as pornographic, condom distribution and the legalizing of prostitution are some examples. On the other hand, it is the churches or religious groups which have occupied the high ground of compassion and caring for the ill and the dying and sheltered those who may have been abandoned and deserted by society.

AIDS as divine retribution

Religion has for centuries been used as a moral justification for homophobic persecution and, by extension, in more recent times AIDS has been held to be the expression of divine anger against this depravity. The combination of reactionary politics and intolerance, which is defended by severe and unbending religious convictions, has been in the forefront of the attacks on the rights of gay people. The oft-quoted passage from Leviticus 20:13 on the death penalty for male homosexual intercourse as well as the plague which destroyed 24 000 of the Children of Israel because of their moral profligacy (Numbers 25:9) are commonly quoted as the biblical sources for the advent of the modern AIDS epidemic.

The pursuit of high-risk activities is a free-will choice. If the individual chooses to flagrantly disobey such a clearly stated biblical prohibition, he must be held to be fully responsible for the consequences to himself. There have been religious apologists who have counter-attacked the proposal that AIDS is a divine retribution by highlighting the plight of the 'innocents' – those who have acquired their infections through no free-will choice of their own – babies, unwitting spouses, blood transfusion recipients, haemophiliacs and health care workers. (This argument becomes even more cogent in developing countries where AIDS has caused devastation on such a vast scale and is so much the result of poverty, social upheaval and uncontrolled urbanization due to famine. The disease here could barely be construed as a punishment for the wrong free-will choice!)

Fortunately, as the epidemic progresses and as experience with the disease becomes more mature, the human mind has been better able to deal with a disease of such awesome proportions and a more reasoned approach is now prevailing. The view of AIDS as a divine punishment is also waning with the relative decline of the epidemic in the male homosexual population.

However, the conflict between religious teachings and values and the measures used to control the epidemic have still remained and the controversies continue unabated, especially in countries where religion plays a dominant role in the culture and the regulation of society.

Conflicts between religion and AIDS control

Clearly, religious teachings and the broad aims of AIDS control to modify high-risk behaviour coincide totally with each other. It is really only in certain selected issues of the means used to effect behavioural change or reduce the chances of transmission that points of dispute have arisen.

Many authorities and workers in the field of AIDS education have frequently decried what they feel to be the overly prudish, vague and coy handling of educational material for AIDS. To be effective, it has been maintained that educational messages need to be forthright, unambiguous and explicit. The more brazen advertising which appeared in response to this often offended and shocked, and resulted in continuing friction between AIDS educationalists and religious spokesmen. But perhaps a more fundamental difficulty is that of the content of much of the AIDS educational material compiled and endorsed by public health authorities which recognizes, and by implication is seen as accepting and even condoning, sexual intercourse outside of marriage and homosexual intercourse.

There is a deep concern within the religious establishments that the recognition and publicizing of activities that are not only directly against the teachings of the faith, but are also those which would lead to the breakdown of family values, are given a tacit 'stamp of approval' by authorities of the state (even though there may be no official stance of support for these activities). There is also a distaste felt in many traditional sections of the community for the gaudy AIDS parades, AIDS fairs and AIDS concerts. While these forms of entertainment aim to use the media of music, dance, spectacle and even humour to put a serious educational message across, the mixing of frivolity and levity with a painful and tragic disease is an affront to many. Unfortunately the conflict tends to widen the rift between two strongly held views, to the detriment of each. Preaching from the pulpit and admonitions from teachers tend to demean and debase the best intentioned of educational programmes and foster an 'us' *versus* 'them' attitude. On the other hand, the scoffing and ridiculing of the religious standpoint serves only to alienate a very significant proportion of the population amongst whose members are many who could still remain vulnerable to behavioural risks and who should be reached by appropriate educational messages. Clearly the only resolution to this difficulty is that due recognition must be given to the diversity of cultural and religious needs of different communities. To be effective and to avoid offence these vastly different viewpoints must be specifically and appropriately targeted in the compiling of educational programmes.

Other facets of AIDS control have caused similar conflicts between what are seen by some as necessary measures to reduce transmission of HIV and by others as a sanctioning of immorality. Some of these issues include the legalizing of prostitution, the providing of facilities for the exchanging of used needles and syringes for new ones and the supplying of condoms to prisoners. Advertising, selling and distribution of condoms have long been a source of difficulty with religious establishments, as has the option of abortion for HIV-infected pregnant women. The AIDS epidemic, which has laid major emphasis on the propagation of condom usage as a powerful weapon in the fight against AIDS and also abortion as a facility to prevent vertically transmitted AIDS, has again brought these old conflicts into the forefront.

With the further advances of the epidemic there will be calls with renewed vigour by fundamentalists for a return to religious prescriptions and to their values of sexual relationships within the bounds of marriage alone, as the only means of controlling the epidemic. These viewpoints deserve to be considered and respected as they have a clear relevance and importance to large sections of the community. The message is unquestionably correct and the wider the community that can put effect to these exhortations, the greater the size of the population which will be protected from HIV infection. There is, however, little relevance in preaching this message to the poor, the destitute and the homeless, where sexual promiscuity is not a free-choice decision but a means of survival. There also seems to be no virtue in the admonishing and castigating type of preaching which serves only further to alienate individuals and foster the counterproductive kind of conflict which threatens effective AIDS control programmes.

Conclusions

The legal and ethical parameters of the AIDS epidemic are constantly evolving and adapting to new circumstances, new issues and new difficulties. The patchwork quilt of the AIDS story is continually being added to and subtracted from by new laws and regulations and new court decisions. A never-ending combination of circumstances has arisen which challenge the existing legal framework and provoke the enactment of yet newer legislation to cope with issues ranging from anti-discrimination in housing and employment, to culpability for transmission of infection and breaches of confidentiality. There is, however, no universal ethic for humankind and ethical frameworks will differ from country to country and ethical practices will also differ from community to community. What is, however, common to all of humankind is that there are reactionary conservative viewpoints and there are also aggressively revolutionary viewpoints. The former would need to be persuaded that pragmatic goals and moral ideals are actually coincidental and that, in the final analysis, the most effective form of control is not to coerce but to convince. The latter viewpoints need to be persuaded that to offend and to provoke serve only to widen existing differences and can only serve to be counterproductive.

The ethical approach to the control of the infection appears to be swinging back to calls for an end to the special considerations enjoyed by AIDS. There is a growing feeling that the so-called 'AIDS exceptionalism' needs to be replaced by a returning of the disease to 'mainstream medicine', and that the traditionalist public health measures for infectious diseases and sexually transmitted diseases should be applied in the same way to AIDS. This is partly the result of a growing alarm at the seeming inability to control the spread of the epidemic by existing measures, partly a result of the waning influence of the gay activist lobby and also partly due to improvements in the prospects of treating the disease itself; for example, the treatment of early asymptomatic infection. One would, however, need to guard against the rush to implement simplistic or 'obvious' solutions. Given the complexities of the social and socio-political ramifications of the disease, the ripple effect of newer control measures needs to be very critically examined before being put into practice.

9

Measuring the dimensions of the AIDS epidemic – AIDS epidemiology

LIVERPOOL
JOHN MOORES UNIVERSITY
AVRIL ROBARTS LRC
TEL. 0151 231 4022

Faced with the vastness of the AIDS epidemic there are many who have paused not only to reflect on the extent and implications of the disease, but also to question the validity of data as well as the accuracy of the monitoring and tracking of the epidemic. AIDS has an enormous reserve of sceptics both on the side of those who insist that the data are under-played, either deliberately by the authorities or unintentionally by scientists (due to inadequate reporting), and on those who ridicule the 'over-exaggeration' of the figures. Media portrayal of AIDS statistics often resembles a roller-coaster with dramatic, panic-mongering figures or alternately down-played and taciturn reporting. Bombarded with such conflicting reports on AIDS, it is hardly surprising that there is such a great deal of confusion on where AIDS is and where AIDS is going.

Undoubtedly, the dimensions of human diseases and human health are difficult to measure. Data on disease are dependent on many variables such as patients seeking medical advice, correct diagnoses being made, the awareness and willingness of the medical attendant to transmit information to a registry, and the resources and abilities of the authorities to process that information.

It is therefore not surprising, given this seemingly insecure basis for the dimensions of human disease in general, that sceptics have not been tardy in questioning whether AIDS is really of recent origin – as is scientifically held. The question must arise as to whether AIDS could not have been in existence for many decades without health authorities being aware of it. Also, what other diseases may be present in humankind which have not yet reached the attention of health authorities. If a new disease similar to

AIDS should arise in the future, how ready would the establishment be to recognize it in the future and how long would the delay period be before it is discovered? If an old disease were to reappear, would it be detected at an early stage? Furthermore, what certainty is there that infections such as smallpox, which was declared to have been eradicated from humankind in 1979, has indeed been totally eradicated?

These and many similar questions emphasize the need to detect and to monitor human diseases as well as to evaluate the effectiveness of the measures that are implemented to control them. These questions fall within the ambit of the science of epidemiology and within the professional expertise of scientists called epidemiologists who function in public health facilities as well as in academic institutions throughout the world. Before considering the epidemiology of AIDS in particular, it would be necessary to first discuss what precisely is meant by the terms 'epidemiology' and 'surveillance' and how this discipline relates to viral diseases in general.

Epidemiology, surveillance and monitoring

The meaning of epidemiology

There is no completely clear and embracing definition of the word 'epidemiology'. The study of epidemics is but a small portion of a very much broader discipline which essentially involves itself with the study of the behaviour and extent of disease in populations, and population factors which affect the characteristics and manifestations of disease. Over recent times, the science of epidemiology has expanded enormously. It now occupies a very substantial part of medical science with some half dozen or so professional journals in the English language solely devoted to the subject. Professional epidemiologists are medically or scientifically trained individuals who plan and execute investigations to glean information on disease and on population characteristics relevant to disease. Infectious causes of disease are but one part, albeit a very substantial part, of the study of epidemiology, which also includes non-infectious causes of morbidity and mortality such as trauma, substance abuse, cigarette smoking, nutrition and cancer.

The term 'surveillance' is used in its epidemiological sense, to denote the process of the systematic recruitment of data about disease and the analysis and processing of these data. Processed information is given to interested parties, including the suppliers of the data, so that they can address the problems of the disease in a meaningful way. Surveillance may be active or passive. Active surveillance involves the deliberate planning of investigations, projects or programmes to obtain data which would otherwise not be available. The term 'passive surveillance' is used to indicate situations where data are being automatically generated as a 'by-product' of other programmes; for example, the various routine screening programmes such as the screening of military recruits and blood donor testing. While these data are already available, it may, of course, still need the effort to retrieve them from computer databases or records and to subsequently analyse and study them. Surveillance may be carried out as a single project or as a regular activity, or it may be carried out on a continual ongoing basis.

(The terms 'active' and 'passive' surveillance are also often used in a different sense by the bodies or institutions whose function it is to collect and process data. Here, active surveillance is used to indicate the deliberate and regular contacting of suppliers of data to recruit the relevant information, whereas 'passive surveillance' is used where reliance is placed on suppliers of the data to remit information on their own accord.)

The term 'monitoring' is used in an epidemiological sense to refer to the long-term continuing surveillance of disease or population characteristics as part of a structured health programme. Generally a monitoring programme would be a formal section of a governmental or non-governmental institution and this would be one of the main ways of closing the 'epidemiological loop'. This 'loop' refers to the essential feedback and response which is the raison d'être for the existence of epidemiology. Thus, the purpose of epidemiology is not only to be able to produce data but, of equal importance, to be able to act on the implications which flow from it. This executive arm of epidemiology could involve an educational component as well as a more active response to institute meaningful interventions to control, reduce or even eliminate the disease.

The terms 'prevalence' and 'incidence' are frequently used to describe the extent of disease and perhaps need to be clarified. The prevalence of a disease indicates the total number of people infected or affected. Point prevalence refers to the number involved at a particular point of time and period prevalence over a duration of time, for example six months or two years. The incidence of a disease means the number of *new* cases of that disease occurring over a period of time, often expressed per annum.

Instruments of surveillance

Disease notification

Physicians or other health care workers may be compelled by law to provide details of diseases seen by themselves during the course of their medical practices. This is called statutory notification. Alternatively, physicians may be requested to provide these details on a voluntary basis – generally referred to as reporting or voluntary reporting. Many pathways for transmitting information are available – mail, telephone, telegram, fax or regular visits by investigating teams. Notification or reporting may or may not make provision for anonymity. The list of statutory notifiable diseases varies from country to country. Diseases which are designated as notifiable are those which pose a threat to public health and which are amenable to effective intervention. These would include formidable epidemic diseases such as rabies, cholera, plague, viral haemorrhagic fevers and also vaccine-preventable diseases such as poliomyelitis and measles, or non-infectious diseases where public health measures can be effectively instituted, such as lead poisoning or exposure to insecticides. In most countries a statutory notifiable disease list would comprise some 20–30 conditions.

Undoubtedly, statutory notification has been of immense value in the control of many conditions, especially infectious diseases. Notification rates are usually good for those diseases which are uncommon, clearly recognizable and are dramatic in their impact; for example, rabies, viral haemorrhagic fever and poliomyelitis. However, with many of the other diseases, for example viral hepatitis, notification rates are abysmally low, and data from notifications are usually of little value. Legal coercion is seldom applied to compel doctors to report notifiable diseases and in some cases monetary rewards are offered as an incentive to notify, but generally with little success.

Associated with statutory notification there are a number of legal instruments and regulations which empower public health authorities to institute measures deemed to be in the interests of public safety; for example, enforced hospitalization, taking of specimens for laboratory investigations, quarantining, forbidding of infected persons working in certain occupations such as food handling and closing down of food establishments.

'Viral watch' programmes

In many parts of the world, networks of 'sentinel' or 'spotter' physicians have been established through their respective professional bodies and associations, to act as gleaners of information about various diseases. A particularly well developed programme which exists in a number of countries is the so-called 'viral watch' programme. The main target diseases that are reported on are viral respiratory illnesses and, together with useful clinical information, the sentinel physicians often also supply valuable specimens for analysis. For example, influenza monitoring is dependent on the viral networks not only to alert the relevant authorities about the appearance and extent of infection, but also to provide material for virus isolation and characterization. This information is used, among others, in the designing of future vaccines. The viral watch network is also frequently used for the monitoring of other virus conditions.

Laboratory results and records

Clinical laboratories are frequently a valuable resource for the reporting of disease and infection. For many of the statutory notifiable conditions laboratory data are used to supplement and sometimes may be the only source of disease notification. Data are also often easy to retrieve from laboratory records – usually a source of relatively unambiguous and clearly defined information.

Hospital/clinic records and death certification

Hospitals and clinics, as with private doctors, have the same responsibility to transmit information regarding notifiable and reportable diseases. In addition, hospital and clinic records are often used retrospectively in surveillance programmes or projects to retrieve information regarding diseases. The value of this resource for the collection of information will become increasingly important as computerization streamlines the tasks of retrieval and collection.

The registrar of births and deaths has long been used as a source of information regarding the prevalence of disease or to chart the extent of epidemics or other health-related events. Although records such as those of hospitals or death certificates have the advantage of easy accessibility, they also have the serious drawback that the reliability of the data depends on the accuracy of the diagnosis which is recorded. Unfortunately this may well be misleading. Frequently the admission diagnosis for a patient entering a hospital may be substantially different from what is eventually diagnosed. Even a discharge diagnosis might reflect one aspect of the patient's final medical condition and omit to mention other aspects of a disease complex which may be more relevant to surveillance. Death certificates are notorious for frequently giving the cause of death as the final event rather than the initial cause of the illness. For example, a patient admitted to hospital with viral hepatitis may subsequently develop pneumonia as a complication and the discharge diagnosis or the diagnosis on the death certificate may be given as pneumonia rather than the viral hepatitis which was the initial cause of the illness.

Serosurveillance

The prevalence of an infectious agent in a population is often computed by determining the proportion of individuals in a representative sample of that population who have antibodies in their serum to the infectious agent, that is surveillance by means of serology, or serosurveillance. With many infectious agents, the presence of antibodies also denotes immunity to an infectious agent and serosurveillance will, at the same time, indicate the proportion of individuals who are immune to the organism, whether the antibodies were due to immunization or a result of having been infected with it (it is usually impossible to distinguish whether the antibodies are from immunization or infection). There are a few infections, of which HIV is perhaps the most important example, where the presence of antibodies does not indicate immunity, but is rather an indication of ongoing infection and infectivity, as discussed in Chapter 3.

Serosurveillance may be active or passive. Thus, it may be carried out as an active pre-planned and deliberate study where specimens are obtained by taking blood from representative groups of individuals. Alternatively, surveillance may be carried out by collecting and analysing data generated by screening programmes already in existence such as blood donor screening, pre-employment screening, or screening of military recruits. Both active and passive serosurveillance have advantages and disadvantages. Active recruitment of samples has the benefit that fresh specimens are obtained and are tested with a technology optimized for the project. Also the selection of the samples to be tested is pre-planned to comply with statistical and other methodological requirements of scientifically planned epidemiological studies. Usually control samples can be obtained which are carefully matched in relevant details to the samples being investigated.

The major drawback of active surveillance projects is the expense involved in collecting specimens and testing them. Also there is usually some degree of bias in the selection of the samples because of the need to rely on volunteers to provide material. In some situations the bias may act in the direction of underestimating the prevalence of an infectious agent because volunteers would tend to be groups from the better informed, higher socio-economic status of society; for example, volunteers drawn from university students and laboratory workers. In other situations the bias could work in overestimating the true prevalence in a population; for example, when the volunteers have a vested personal interest to be tested because they know they are in a higher than average risk group. This is a particular problem with HIV testing.

An additional problem with active surveillance is that these projects can, ethically, only be carried out on adults and with many infectious diseases it is of great importance to establish at what age infection starts becoming important. Alternative methods of obtaining blood specimens other than from the vein (venepuncture) are being increasingly utilized because of their convenience and also because they may well be ethically more acceptable, especially with regard to obtaining specimens from children. These include capillary blood, where a drop of blood produced by pricking the finger or the heel of a small baby is allowed to be drawn into a fine hollow glass capillary tube. This capillary tube can then be sealed off with clay and sent to a laboratory for testing. A more convenient way of testing capillary blood is to allow it to drop onto a piece of absorbent filter paper. The dried blood spot can then be sent to a laboratory where it is allowed to soak in a small test tube of buffer solution to dissolve out the immunoglobulins for subsequent antibody testing. Dried blood spots on filter paper can be easily transported once they are sealed in a plastic bag containing a desiccant, and can even be sent in the mail. A still easier and more convenient way of obtaining a specimen for antibody testing, which is especially applicable to serosurveillance involving children, is the use of saliva as a testing specimen (Chapter 5).

Passive serosurveillance has, of course, the advantage that it is far cheaper to carry out and consequently much larger numbers can be analysed. For example, serological data banks involving information on literally hundreds of thousands of donors annually are automatically generated on a continual basis because the tests are carried out routinely for screening purposes and usually are accompanied by good documentation with each of the specimens. The costs involved in the collecting and transporting of the specimens as well as the testing are avoided, and the results are provided with relatively little effort. The big disadvantage of passive serosurveillance is that there is total reliance on the sampling method which happened to have been used (this would not be a difficulty with the large numbers involved in blood donor testing), and also, sometimes, the testing techniques which are used in the routine tests. Frequently there is considerable bias with many of the populations sampled; for example, voluntary blood donors represent only a particular segment of society, usually a more socially responsible, lower-risk population. In addition, many infectious agents which are of importance to public health are not tested for in routine screening programmes, and an active project would have to be carried out to obtain information on the prevalence of those infections.

A strategy for prevalence studies which is intermediate between active and passive serosurveillance makes use of serum banks. Many laboratories and scientific institutions maintain banks of serum samples stored in freezers. If adequately catalogued, these banks are an extremely important resource of material which can be retrieved and examined for the presence of antibodies to a particular infectious agent. They obviate the expense and difficulty of collecting specimens yet, if the bank is sufficiently large, it still allows for the same pre-planning in the make-up of the groups of specimens to be tested, as in the case of an active serosurveillance project. Serum specimens can be stored virtually indefinitely in freezers and, provided thawing and refreezing is kept to a minimum, the level of antibodies does not deteriorate significantly. (These serum banks have been of great value for tracing back in history when infections first appeared in humans or to investigate the nature and possible causal agents responsible for epidemics in years gone past. This has spawned a discipline of its own called sero-archeology.)

Pitfalls in surveillance and interpretation of data

The science of epidemiology and its related discipline of statistics have established stringent rules for the correct, reliable and accurate computation of data on disease and related health issues. The collection and processing of data are fraught with pitfalls and sources of error. Amongst the more important and commoner errors are sampling or unsatisfactory matching of controls for comparative studies.

To look for the prevalence of a particular phenomenon such as infection or immunity in a population it is, of course, impossible to test the entire population. A sample must be selected which is large enough to encompass the variety which would be present in the population and also sufficiently representative of the population. To avoid bias the sample must be adequately randomized. Frequently samples from a population are too small (often dictated by costs and logistic difficulties in getting enough specimens) or are inadequately representative (they may tend to have a greater proportion of a particular type of individual than is actually present in the population). It must be noted that the term 'population' may also be used to denote a subset thereof, who share a characteristic, such as children or adults or elderly individuals, or groups of a defined age, or gender, or race, or people pursuing a particular activity or a socio-economic stratum, and so on. The term 'sample' is used for the group of individuals who are actually tested and who are deemed to be representative of the population from which they were derived.

In comparative studies, it becomes necessary to compare the sample under investigation with another sample which needs to be matched in every detail, for example age, race and socio-economic status, other than for the particular factors that are being investigated. Imperfectly matched controls are a frequent source of error in these kinds of studies.

The executive arm of epidemiology

The collection of information on the health and disease status of the population is a costly exercise and really can only be justified if there is the capability for an effective response to control, reduce or even eliminate a threat to public health. The effector arm which responds to epidemiological information is obviously as important a component as that which collects and processes data.

The appropriate response by national and international public health authorities may take various forms depending on the individual situation. It may involve an immunization campaign; for example, an influenza vaccine campaign to contend with an imminent threat of a major influenza epidemic or a mass poliomyelitis immunization campaign if cases of paralytic poliomyelitis are detected, or mass immunization against yellow fever in an endemic zone when there is a flare up of infection. On the basis of epidemiological data the response may well be that of a recommendation for routine immunization where there is widespread evidence of significant infection; for example, hepatitis B immunization in Africa and Asia, or Japanese encephalitis in the Far East. Information on endemic infectious diseases is of importance to international travellers to enable them to be immunized before entering affected countries; for example, yellow fever, Japanese encephalitis or for prophylaxis against malaria.

Epidemiological information permits national and international authorities to impose regulations such as statutory notification, quarantine and international travel regulations. National and international surveillance publications such as the *WHO Weekly Epidemiological Record*, the *Mortality and Morbidity Weekly Report* of the CDC and the *Communicable Diseases Record* of the Communicable Diseases Surveillance Centre in the UK, as well as many others, are widely circulated and interchanged between countries. The majority of these surveillance bulletins are freely available on the Internet. In addition a variety of epidemiology bulletin boards, discussion groups and e-mail lists have sprung up to rapidly disseminate information regarding epidemics to professionals and to public health authorities.

On rare occasions public health responses have been damaging. For instance, an alert by the CDC in 1976 of an impending return of swine influenza (which caused the devastating pandemic of 1918) resulted in the President of the USA issuing a directive for a nationwide influenza immunization campaign. After some 20 million doses of vaccine were administered, the immunization campaign was abruptly halted when epidemiological surveillance began implicating the vaccine in the causation of a paralytic condition called the Guillain-Barré syndrome. Subsequent studies have, however, totally exonerated the influenza vaccine from causing this condition. However, both debacles, the misjudged panic response leading to a nationwide immunization campaign as well as the subsequent incorrect aspersions of the influenza vaccine, are some examples of the more negative results of epidemiological surveillance.

Epidemiological methodology in the AIDS epidemic

The methodologies used for the collection of information on diseases in general are employed in a similar way for the collection of data on AIDS and HIV infection. There are, however, some difficulties which are peculiar or even unique to AIDS. Amongst these are the great variations in the prevalence of the infection in different populations and the difficulties this imposes in getting samples that are sufficiently representative of all the people of a country. The long incubation period of AIDS, that is the time from asymptomatic infection to clinical disease, is a cause of many errors and inaccuracies, especially the under-recognition of infection. Perhaps the greatest problem in the collection of adequate data on the disease is related to the social and personal gravity of a diagnosis of HIV infection. This causes unprecedented fears not only of being tested but also that the results are accessible in the records of a laboratory or an institute.

In spite of these difficulties, it was the vigilance of the monitoring machinery of the CDC and other public health bodies, as well as the alertness of the physicians who first became aware of the unusual nature of the unfolding epidemic, that initially led to the discovery of the AIDS epidemic in 1980 and 1981. A similar alertness amongst physicians in Europe led to the uncovering of the vast epidemic of HIV infection in sub-Saharan Africa in 1983. It is also these selfsame bodies and institutions, together with their reporting networks, which continually provide the information on the progress of the epidemic.

Factors facilitating HIV and AIDS surveillance

One of the major factors which facilitates HIV surveillance is the high profile which it has both amongst the medical profession and the lay public. The need to convey information regarding a case of HIV or of AIDS is more likely to be foremost in the mind of the attending physician, unlike the situation with some more 'obscure' or 'mundane' conditions which the majority of doctors are not even aware are on the notifiable diseases list.

The high public profile of AIDS has also caused a correspondingly high public motivation and, in turn, a high political motivation to commit funds and resources to AIDS, including those for its surveillance. In most countries funding of AIDS and HIV surveillance is generally more readily forthcoming than for other infectious diseases.

Also facilitating AIDS surveillance is the fact that most AIDS cases, certainly in developed countries, are generally treated in the larger and more sophisticated hospitals. In these facilities, diagnostic resources would be optimal and motivation and awareness of procedures for reporting or notification of cases would be considerably better than in smaller facilities.

Factors hindering HIV and AIDS surveillance

On balance, the difficulties of HIV and AIDS surveillance are considerably greater and it is these difficulties which make the epidemiology of the disease such a particularly challenging exercise.

The enormous fear that individuals have, not only for the testing and its implications, but also for the fact that the results of the test could be on permanent record at the laboratory, has resulted in huge difficulties in the design and interpretation of surveillance studies. The planning and execution of AIDS and HIV surveillance programmes and projects are dominated by issues of confidentiality and the preservation of anonymity, which have not infrequently led to conflicts between the interests of high-risk groups and those of health authorities wishing to carry out surveillance studies. In many parts of the world gay activist groups have actively campaigned against the HIV test. In societies of a lesser degree of sophistication and education, fear and superstition usually fanned by grotesque distortions of the implications of a positive HIV diagnosis have greatly compounded the difficulties in obtaining samples, particularly from those very groups where the urgency for HIV investigation is even greater.

Further difficulties in HIV surveillance are related to the peculiar characteristics of the infection itself. The extraordinarily long 'silent' period of infection means that for every clinically apparent case there is a vast, but variably sized, iceberg of concealed infection. This means that there are, in reality, two separate components of the epidemiological challenge – firstly, to determine how reliable the number of visible peaks of the iceberg are and, secondly, to determine the size of the concealed portion of the iceberg. Unfortunately, the extent to which 'silent' HIV infection is detectable or is able to be calculated varies considerably between different countries and also between groups within a country. Furthermore the silently infected individual is important not only as a statistic but also because he or she may well be a source of further transmission to non-infected individuals at a rate which, by nature, is highly variable.

The capabilities of response

The response to the striking epidemiology of AIDS should by rights be particularly powerful and effective. There is obviously little lack of public resolve or government will to fight the AIDS epidemic and to commit resources or funds to whatever needs to be addressed. Indeed, it is quite often the zealousness in responding to the AIDS epidemic, which has some-times led to the diversion of resources away from other health programmes, that has come under criticism, especially in poorer countries with limited health budgets.

Nevertheless, the response to the epidemiology of AIDS has been severely restricted by several factors. Firstly, the tools available to respond are very limited. There is no effective vaccine and no curative drug. Preventive options which do exist are those which are perceived to be directed to the limiting of a human being's most basic pleasures. Reduction of sexual part-ners, safe sex practices and use of condoms are not readily accepted by individuals who are at risk precisely because of these practices. On occa-sion, unfortunately not too infrequently, confrontation has occurred between groups who have been marginalized by society (such as homosexual men) and the health authorities, or between minority inner-city populations and officialdom. Furthermore, the political response to public pressure has, all too often, been discriminatory legislation and regulations which serve to drive the wedge in even further.

One of the major contributing factors to the spread of HIV has been the common combination of despair, poverty, crime, prostitution and drug abuse. The addressing of these broad social ills which stem primarily from economic hardship is considerably broader than HIV control specifically. How effective the measures to control the HIV epidemic are would be difficult to assess because of the vast iceberg of concealed infection. New cases of AIDS would still continue to be manifested even if there were to be no new infections. In fact, the rate of development of new cases of AIDS would barely be affected for a few years, as the vast majority of these AIDS cases would be the result of HIV infection contracted some years previously.

Specific problems of AIDS epidemiology in developing countries

However difficult the collection, processing and response to AIDS data is in the developed world, these problems are vastly magnified in the developing world. The gross inadequacy of health care facilities alone will ensure that only a fraction of AIDS cases ever get reported. Laboratory facilities for the diagnosis of HIV infection or of the opportunistic infections are similarly few and far between and formal structures to collect and analyse epidemiological data are markedly deficient. In addition to all of this is the major problem, seen so commonly in Africa, of patients reporting for medical attention at a very late stage of the disease due to the competing influences of practitioners of alternate medicine, especially the traditional healers, as well as cultural and economic barriers to access to western medicine.

The capabilities for response to the AIDS epidemic in the developing world is correspondingly poor. Socio-economic hardships have contributed greatly to the acceleration of HIV transmission. Vast population migrations from rural areas into the urban conglomerates of the Third World have spawned a massive problem of uncontrolled urbanization which has been even further aggravated in the African continent by drought and famine. Enormous squatter camps with hopelessly inadequate facilities and extreme overcrowding have exacerbated the poverty and also its bedfellow, prostitution.

Another feature of many of the cities of the developing world is the single-sex hostels – the huge structures housing migrant labourers who are separated for long periods from their families in the countryside – and the attendant female prostitution industry that they spawn. The difficulties in advocating a reduction in sex partners to women whose alternative is starvation and who are, in addition, culturally unempowered to negotiate any conditions for sexual intercourse, such as the use of condoms, are hardly less than those of the men forced by economic realities to work in cities and separated from their regular sexual partners.

Cultural influences have often been responsible for a somewhat more resigned attitude to AIDS and its lethality than is the case in the West. Also AIDS is often not perceived to be a sexually transmitted diseases as it rarely manifests itself, as lesions in the genital tract, and this is not infrequently a barrier to efforts to change sexual habits. In a continent beset with massive health priorities such as malnutrition, tuberculosis, gastro-enteritis and measles, AIDS is often seen as yet another health issue to be dealt with in its turn.

The global status of AIDS

Reported and notified AIDS data

The data which form the cornerstone of AIDS epidemiology are those of reported and notified AIDS. The cumulative number of AIDS cases reported throughout the world is published bi-annually in a publication of the World Health Organization called the *Weekly Epidemiological Record*. In its publication of 28 November 1997, the total number of cases reported cumulatively in the world up to that date was 1 736 958, of which some 48.3% (839 189) were reported from the Americas, 35.5% (617 463) from Africa, 11.4% (197 374) from Europe, 4.3% (74 431) from Asia and 0.5% (8 501) from Oceania.

As important as AIDS figures are, a number of major reservations should be borne in mind in evaluating them. There are, indeed, a number of striking anomalies in these figures. For example, the greatest pool of infection is known to be in sub-Saharan Africa (almost two-thirds of all HIV-infected individuals in the world). Yet only about a third of all reported AIDS cases come from that continent. Another equally striking anomaly is that pertaining to the Asian continent which houses over half of humankind, yet has only reported 4.3% of all AIDS cases. How complete are these reported figures and how well do they measure the extent of the epidemic?

The definition of AIDS, as mentioned in Chapter 1, has undergone a number of changes over the years to improve on its specificity (that is, its ability to avoid diagnosing as AIDS clinically similar conditions which are not AIDS) as well as its sensitivity (that is, its ability to pick up as many AIDS cases as possible with the clinical criteria which comprise the definition). In countries which have poor health care facilities and few diagnostic resources and where the prevalence of HIV is still low, there is some evidence that a certain proportion of cases are falsely diagnosed as AIDS. Other than this, there is generally no major problem in overdiagnosis of AIDS cases. The error in AIDS reporting is rather in the direction of underdiagnosis and underreporting. Underdiagnosis of AIDS is due to the defining criteria being too insensitive to register those cases which may have reached the stage of AIDS in terms of the course of the disease, but where the patient does not display all of the clinical criteria needed for the strict definition of the disease and is therefore not recorded as an AIDS case. A more significant cause of error is underreporting. The calculation of the extent of underreporting is difficult and is based on the comparison of the reported figures to the figures obtained by an alternative technique which is used to validate these reported figures. These calculations have estimated that the degree of underreporting in the USA can vary from 0 to 45% while in the UK it is somewhat better at 5–20%. In Africa underreporting is estimated to be up to 90%.

Delays in the reporting of AIDS cases to national registries is a variable cause of underestimating the total number of cases in developed countries. In developing countries the reporting of the number of AIDS cases to the WHO is often seriously out of date. For example, in the WHO report of AIDS data at 28 November 1997, figures supplied by some countries dated back to December 1990. In countries where the epidemic has only relatively recently been established, the number of reported AIDS cases may very significantly undervalue the extent of infection. Thus, in the early stages of an epidemic, the number of HIV-infected individuals is over a hundred times the number of reported AIDS cases. As the epidemic advances the ratio of HIV to AIDS may drop to 10 to 1 or less. The extraordinarily low number of AIDS cases in some Asian countries (for example, only 155 cases reported from China) may be partly explained on the basis of the epidemic having only relatively recently been introduced into the continent. Therefore, the true extent of the HIV epidemic in the population is more precisely represented by the prevalence of HIV infection or the total number of HIV-infected persons.

Determinations of the extent of HIV infection

The number of individuals infected with HIV can be calculated from the figure of reported AIDS cases, although the accuracy of this estimation would be dependent on the reliability of AIDS reporting or notification. This back-calculation method is based on the ratio of AIDS cases to HIV infection. However, as mentioned above, this ratio decreases with the length of time that the epidemic has been in existence in the country and the incubation period correspondingly decreases with the length of time of the HIV epidemic in a country. The incubation period, therefore, needs to be built into this back-calculation.

The second method of calculating the extent of HIV infection is by determining the prevalence of infection in different sentinel population groups. Because the prevalence of HIV is far from being randomly distributed, a number of groups of individuals are used as sentinels, to represent the spectrum of risk activities in a population. This so-called 'family of serosurveys' usually consists of some passive surveillance programmes, for example prospective blood donors, who represent the lowest risk group, and also some active surveillance studies, for example mothers attending antenatal clinics (representing a more or less average risk group of sexually active individuals), tuberculosis patients (representing a higher risk group) and high-risk groups such as attenders of sexually transmitted diseases clinics. Provided that the sentinel groups are sufficiently representative of the spectrum of risk activities in a population, the total number of people infected can be calculated from the estimated total numbers belonging to each of the groups sampled.

Virtually all countries in the world carry out some kind of serosurveillance in their populations. The value of these studies depends on how carefully they have been designed. Statistical pre-planning is essential to ensure that the sample sizes are adequate and are randomly chosen to be sufficiently representative of the population. One of the major problems in surveillance studies is the bias which applies to any sampling design. Testing may be done on a compulsory, voluntary or anonymous basis. Compulsory testing will impose a bias on the results as it is the high-risk individuals who will be more likely to attempt to escape being tested and this could cause a falsely low prevalence figure. Participation bias could similarly affect the validity of voluntary testing. In some situations of voluntary testing the prevalence figure may be falsely high as the individuals who are more likely to volunteer would be those who are at higher risk or have had an exposure which has caused them sufficient anxiety to persuade them to come for testing. Alternately, it may be falsely low if high-risk individuals are more reticent to volunteer for testing because of fear of accidental or unauthorised disclosure of the results.

Anonymous testing may be carried out in two ways – anonymous linked and anonymous unlinked. In linked anonymous testing, the identity of the specimen is unknown to the laboratory so that the confidentiality of the person is preserved. However, the specimen does carry an identifying number and individual results could be retrieved from the laboratory by using this number. Confidentiality, however, cannot be totally guaranteed, as the results of a particular individual could be obtained by collusion between the clinic and the laboratory. This fear of a potential breakdown of confidentiality could cause the same participation bias as with the voluntary testing strategy. The least degree of bias occurs in unlinked anonymous screening. Here, all identifying labels or signs are removed from the specimen tubes so that there is no way a result can be traced back to an individual and confidentiality is guaranteed. This strategy has the drawback that it is of no value in finding cases of HIV for follow-up and counselling.

Nevertheless, it is the optimal method, from an epidemiological point of view, for obtaining as unbiased and representative a sample as possible.

Globally, the WHO had estimated that, at the end of 1991, there were some eight to ten million infected adults; in the Americas there were estimated to have been two million infections up to that date (one million in North America and one million in Latin America), some half a million infections in Western Europe, in sub-Saharan Africa, six million adults, and in South and Southeast Asia (particularly India and Thailand), over one million infections. By the end of 1997, the global estimate of people living with HIV/AIDS had increased to 30.6 million. This increase was, however, uneven. In the Americas the estimate had increased to only 2.47 million and in Europe scarcely increased at all – to 530 000; in contrast, the estimate for sub-Saharan Africa increased over threefold, to 20.8 million, while that for South and Southeast Asia increased sixfold to six million. The impact of these prevalence figures is even more dramatic if they are expressed in relation to the total population; for example, in a number of urban populations of central and southern Africa, the prevalence of HIV is calculated to be between 1 in 10 to 1 in 3 of all sexually active adults. In the entire sub-Saharan African adult population, the prevalence is now estimated to be approximately 1 in 40. Clearly these striking figures convey a very dramatic and desperate picture of the extent of the epidemic.

The dynamics of the AIDS epidemic

Trends plotted over a number of years for both AIDS as well as HIV figures have been the bedrock of the evaluation of the dynamics of the epidemic.

A term commonly used to describe the rate of expansion of the epidemic is the doubling time, which means simply the duration of time taken for the number of cases to double. For example, the doubling time of the epidemic in sexually active adults in Africa has been estimated at one to three years in some areas, and as long as five years in less affected areas.

Trend analyses based on HIV prevalence figures have revealed a great deal of information regarding the dynamics of HIV transmission in different parts of the world. For example, in Europe and North America the epidemic curve, which rose sharply in the early 1980s with the explosive outbreak in sexually active homosexual men and intravenous drug abusers, peaked in the mid 1980s, and the incidence of new cases has now dropped significantly. This probably reflects the success of efforts to modify behaviour patterns and reduce high-risk activities. However, there is now a continuing steady increase in the incidence of heterosexually transmitted infection.

In sub-Saharan Africa, the infection started its expansion somewhat later than in North America and is still continuing to rise. The trend in Latin America looks similar although the annual incidence is somewhat lower than in sub-Saharan Africa. In Asia, where the prevalence of infection has been so remarkably low, AIDS is still only at the incipient stage of epidemic spread in some parts such as China and Japan, but is expanding very rapidly in Thailand and India. The annual incidence is expected to continue rising and could overtake that of Africa during the late 1990s and still continue rising into early in the twenty-first century.

Studies of trends in micro-populations have similarly provided extremely important knowledge on HIV behaviour. A striking example of the explosive increase in HIV transmission was observed in prostitutes in Nairobi where the prevalence of infection rose from 4% in 1981 to 61% in 1985 and 90% in 1988. Similarly, sharp increases were seen in a completely different epidemiological milieu, that of intravenous drug abusers in Edinburgh and Milan where, in the early to mid-1980s, the prevalence rose from 5% to 50% in two to three years. In Asian countries, which had reported so few AIDS cases up until the mid-1990s, major expansions of the epidemic are now being experienced, as evidenced by the sixfold increase in continental estimates from 1992 to 1997 as well as data coming from a number of micro-population studies in selected high-risk groups. For example, in India a study in the state of Manipur found no HIV-positive infections in September 1989 and after intensive searching came up with one positive blood sample. By June of the following year 54% of a sample of some 1500 intravenous drug abusers were positive. Similarly, in Thailand and Myanmar, the prevalence of infection in intravenous drug abusers increased from zero to 50% in the space of three to four years. Studies on prostitutes in a number of countries in Southeast Asia have, likewise, recently shown sharp increases in prevalence.

Forecasting the future

The vast implications of the AIDS epidemic to the economic growth of countries, developed as well as developing, has forced scientists into constructing future scenarios for the disease, both for the short-term as well as for the long-term future. Unfortunately, this need for knowledge about what the future holds has also attracted a large number of pseudo-experts who make their own forecasts, often of the distant future, often with a considerable degree of sensationalism and seldom with much scientific basis. For example, a common error in forecasting is the use of doubling times to simply double up on the number of HIV or AIDS cases thus reaching enormously high figures in a number of years (theoretically repeated doubling of any percentage eventually reaches 100%). It must be emphasized that the doubling time is a useful estimation of the *past* history of an epidemic, but cannot be used for future projections of an epidemic as the future growth of epidemic diseases is dependent on many complex factors which often differ substantially from those present in the development of the epidemic up to that date, as will be discussed below.

Epidemics of infectious diseases, both acute and chronic, follow to a greater or lesser extent pre-defined behaviour patterns which can be mathematically charted and, to some extent, predicted. The HIV epidemic, with its particularly long incubation period, its life-long infectivity and its low but unpredictable transmissibility, imposes additional difficulties in forecasting and projecting into the future. For example, one of the fundamental weaknesses in all forecasting methods is that they rely on what has taken place in the past in terms of transmissibility and in terms of the susceptibility of the population, in order to make calculations for the future behaviour of the epidemic. Epidemics initially preferentially involve those individuals who are at higher risk of exposure and who have the greatest degree of susceptibility. The epidemic curve then progressively flattens out and declines as the number of susceptible individuals decreases because those who have already been infected and have recovered generally become immune. In addition the risk of exposure to the agent decreases as the epidemic matures. Eventually, when a sufficient number of individuals in that population are immune (as a result of infection or immunization), the epidemic will die out as there are not enough susceptible individuals for the infection to be transmitted and for the epidemic to be sustained. When that level, or proportion, of individuals in a population who are immune to an agent is reached, that population is said to have herd immunity. With HIV, however, many of the factors of relevance to other infectious diseases are not applicable. For example, there is no recovery or subsequent immunity to HIV infection (nor, of course, is there any vaccine to provide immunity). Furthermore, unlike most other infectious diseases where the ability to transmit infection is temporary and the disease may be clinically obvious, HIV infectivity is presumably permanent and life-long and present mostly during the silent clinical phase. It is not known whether the concept of herd immunity is, in fact, at all applicable to HIV infection. Certainly, with HIV, what can be predicted and even computed is that the proportion of susceptible individuals in terms of risk of exposure will progressively decline as it is the high-risk persons who are the ones who are initially

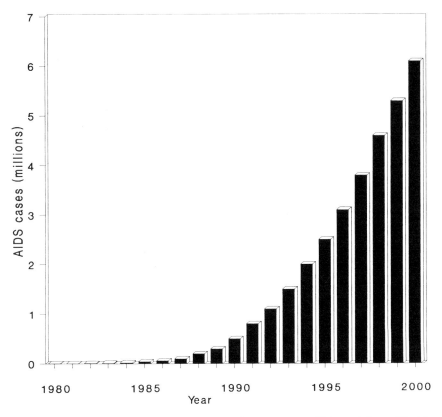

Fig. 9.1 Delphi projection of AIDS cases to the year 2000. (Adapted from *Weekly Epidemiological Record*, No. 30, 28 July 1989, p. 230, with permission from the WHO.)

infected and as the epidemic advances in time there are more and more low-risk individuals left behind. A further unpredictable factor is the effectiveness of intervention programmes and behavioural modifications on the transmissibility of infection.

A number of projection methodologies for HIV have been devised. One of the earliest of these techniques is that of extrapolation. The parameters of the HIV epidemic are plotted and the tendencies which have been displayed up to that time are then extended into the future. Modifications to this extension are made to take into account the progressive decline in population susceptibility, the long incubation period and the reducing ratio of HIV to AIDS cases.

One of the most widely used methods for forecasting AIDS cases is the

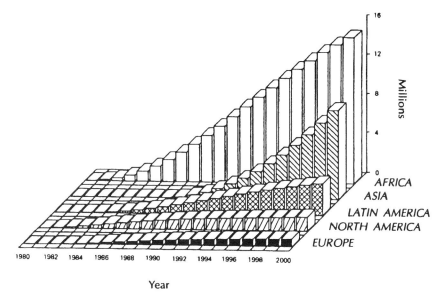

Fig 9.2 Projected cumulative HIV infections in different continents. (Adapted from *Weekly Epidemiological Record*, No 48, 29 November 1991, p. 355, with permission from the WHO).

back-calculation method mentioned previously. This statistical procedure has to rely on the validity and accuracy of reported AIDS figures as well as a knowledge of the incubation time from HIV infection to AIDS. The calculation is carried out as a two-step procedure – back-calculating from the number of AIDS cases to obtain the total pool of HIV-infected individuals and then utilizing the incubation periods to project forward in order to determine the number of future AIDS cases.

Both the extrapolation as well as the back calculation methods are only reliable for short-term prediction of up to a few years.

There are, in addition, techniques that are dependent on mathematical and statistical calculations and also dozens of computer models. Some are based on micro-simulation where variables applicable to individuals or small groups are built into the programme, whereas others are macro-simulation models, which create future scenarios around large populations and national data.

Perhaps the best known of the future projection techniques is that devised by the WHO, called the Delphi projections (Figs. 9.1 and 9.2). The Delphi method relies on the judgement of experts in the field of AIDS with experience in both developed and developing countries, to independently forecast the future of the AIDS epidemic. A Delphi exercise carried out in 1989 involved 14 experts and took place in two stages. In the first stage each of the experts, whose identity was kept secret from the others, independently gave his forecast of AIDS up to the year 2000 in response to a standardized questionnaire. The results were analysed and distributed to each of the participants, but still maintaining the secrecy of the panel. To obtain consensus the participants were then asked to complete a second questionnaire and these were then correlated to produce the Delphi projections.

The WHO estimated the total number of HIV-infected persons at the end of 1997 to be 30.6 million. This figure has already reached the conservative projection of 30–40 million men, women and children for the year 2000. The total number of reported AIDS cases as at the end of 1997 was 1.74 million and was predicted to increase, on average, by a million per year until the year 2000. The majority of these AIDS cases will occur irrespective of how effective any HIV prevention programmes are, as these AIDS cases would be the terminal results of HIV infection already acquired over the last decade.

10

Conclusion: outlook for the future

The electronic media and, perhaps more especially, the print media have often in a very dramatic way reinforced the anxieties and the fears of the 'person in the street' as well as given prematurely false hopes about drugs and vaccine 'breakthroughs'. As the AIDS epidemic approaches the third decade there are now very few people who remain indifferent to this disease. Reflecting one pole of opinion, there is no shortage of shrill banner headlines which eagerly paint a doomsday scenario. 'AIDS set to devastate economy', 'Large parts of the African continent will be depopulated by AIDS', 'The death of Africa?' are but some of the more rampaging headlines. The opposite pole of opinion on AIDS is also occasionally published, such as that of the eminent historian Paul Johnson, in the *Spectator*, London, 1991 – '. . . there are many other areas where money is not only more urgently required, but could be more profitably spent. To divert it into the bottomless pit of AIDS is wicked. What the whole subject requires is a long thoughtful silence'.

How is humankind to deal with this latter day plague? Throughout the ages vast epidemics of infectious diseases have decimated large segments of the human population. Smallpox and then measles carved a swathe of destruction in ancient Rome and then moved into Europe from where they were both carried westward into the New World by the Spanish explorers. The population of the indigenous Indians of Central and South America dropped from an estimated 130 million to about 1.6 million, more as a result of these two infectious diseases than from war. In the nineteenth century measles has been held to have been responsible for the total annihilation of the Indian population of the island of Tierra del Fuego. Plague, the 'Black Death', swept through Europe in the second pandemic of the fourteenth century destroying a quarter of Europe's population. Yellow fever, the curse of the Ancient Mariner and dreaded by sailors and travellers to the tropical world, killed some 20 000 of the 50 000 Europeans living in Central America in the nineteenth century. The huge influenza pandemic of 1918/1919 caused global devastation and some 20 million deaths.

The experience of AIDS is, however, a novel one to mankind. Major epidemics have, until now, been acute infections which certainly exacted a terrible toll in human lives but all were temporary, and when a certain number of individuals had been infected and the population had developed herd immunity, the epidemic would die out. Those who had survived would be immune for life. All of these plagues of yesteryear are now preventable by vaccines or curable by drugs. The mastery over epidemic infectious diseases had seemed all but complete in an age of rapid development of antibiotics and antimicrobials and high technology vaccine manufacture. Never before has humankind been faced with a major epidemic of a slow and prolonged infectious disease with no individual or herd immunity, where the extent of disease so grossly belies the extent of the epidemic of infection, where there is no vaccine or cure and where the control options that are available are so bedevilled by overwhelming social, political, cultural and economic difficulties.

Statistics on AIDS are often bewildering. Sometimes they would suggest a disease of serious, yes, but not critical proportions. For example the cumulative number of AIDS cases over the last 25 years reported to the WHO up to 28 November 1997 was 1 736 958, and is still overshadowed by the annual death tolls of other infectious diseases – 2-3 million each for tuberculosis, diarrhoeal disease and malaria.

At other times statistics on AIDS are alarming, especially those coming from sub-Saharan Africa where less than 10% of the world's population is responsible for some 60% of all HIV infections. Furthermore, that one-fortieth of all adults in this part of the world are infected with a terminal disease, and that each of these individuals can, in turn, act as a fount of infection for yet further spread clearly indicates an epidemic of towering proportions. HIV prevalence figures which do emanate from the African continent are indeed staggering. Some are based on scientific studies which indicate that up to one-third of all sexually active adults living in regions of sub-Saharan Africa are already infected, up to 40% of all women attending antenatal clinics in certain urban centres are HIV positive and therefore that about 1 in 10 to 1 in 5 children born in these parts of the world will be actively infected with the virus and will be dead before having reached their fifth birthday. In addition, more than twice as many non-infected children have been orphaned as a result of AIDS. The prevalence of infection in blood donor populations in some of these countries is 29%, giving a recipient a greater than 1 in 4 chance of being infected per unit of blood if that blood is not screened. The prevalence in female prostitutes in many of the large African cities is close to saturation (up to 90% or even more). Several reports from anecdotal sources have claimed that the prevalence of HIV infection in young military recruits in several African countries is now well over 50%, and in long distance truck drivers who ply their routes through central and southern Africa the prevalence could be closer to 70%.

The measurable costs to humanity of the AIDS epidemic are already immense. In the USA, AIDS has, over the last decade, reversed the declining death rate in men aged 25–44. Thus, between 1970 and 1983, death rates fell from 300 per 100000 to 212 per 100000 in this population. However, they started increasing again after 1983 to reach 236 per 100000 in 1987 and were projected to reach 300 per 100000 by the mid-1990s according to the WHO model. By the late 1980s AIDS had become the leading cause of death in both men and women in the age group 25–34 in New York City.

In sub-Saharan Africa AIDS has already leapt to the prime position as a cause of death in a continent already beset with staggering health burdens. In most countries of the continent AIDS is the leading cause of adult death and in some studies, for example women of child-bearing age in Rwanda, HIV disease was responsible for 90% of deaths. The effect of AIDS on population growth in Africa is controversial. In a number of the earlier long-term projection studies, forecasts of a reversal of population growth were predicted, and some of the less scientific journalistic soothsayers painted doomsday pictures of the depopulation of huge tracts of African soil. However, more recent modelling studies have indicated that the population will continue to grow, although at a significantly reduced rate. Thus, in Africa, the predicted 70 million HIV cases over the next 25 years will be responsible for a reduction of population by 50 million individuals as a direct result of AIDS. The disease would also be responsible for reversing the trend of longer life expectancy; this has now been predicted to be reduced by up to 12 years.

In addition, the infant mortality rate which, with considerable effort from international health authorities, had finally started to show signs of responding to intensive efforts in increasing immunization coverage, is also showing evidence of reversals of erstwhile downward trends, due to the

effects of AIDS. Infant mortality rates have been projected to increase by
10% and childhood mortality by 15%.

There is little comfort from these figures for the callous viewpoint that
AIDS should be looked on as a 'mixed blessing', being a natural way of
addressing the Malthusian nightmare of overpopulation. In fact, the reverse
may well be true. Population trends could actually increase instead of
decrease in response to rising mortality of young adults and children, as
is characteristically seen in socio-economically deprived countries where
high fecundity overcompensates for population losses due to malnutrition
and infectious diseases.

Over and above the impact on mortality, the devastation of AIDS does
have and will have a massive impact on the costs to the health care system
specifically and also to the global economy generally. In the USA the average life-time cost of treating an AIDS patient has been estimated to be about
$70 000, while the total federal bill for HIV in 1992 was estimated to be
$4.3 billion, representing, at that time, some 1.6% of all health-related
costs in the USA.

The costs of AIDS to developing countries such as those in Africa are
not measurable on the same scale as those of developed countries such as
the USA. The cost of treating 100 patients with AIDS in the USA is greater
than the entire health budget of a majority of sub-Saharan African countries. The cost of treating an AIDS patient in Africa has been estimated to
be $150–400 compared with an average per capita expenditure on health
of $15. In some of these countries AIDS treatment may be the equivalent
of up to 4% of the gross national product, which is already in a state of
decline in many countries as a result of the ravages of drought and war.
Aggravating the economic plight even further is the greater likelihood for
the virus to preferentially infect the educated and economically more
productive young men in the community, those with greater disposable
incomes who are able to pursue more active sexual lifestyles. Involvement
of women has similarly devastating economic implications, as they form the
bulk of the agricultural workforce on which many African economies are
so dependent. The growing problem of AIDS orphans in Africa, currently
estimated to be well over 2 million but projected to exceed 10 million by
the end of the 1990s, will be responsible for an even greater load on the
existing meagre facilities of the state and on care-taking facilities, and yet
further reduce available human resources for agriculture and other economic
developments.

A worst case scenario

As discussed in the previous chapter, future predictions of the course of the HIV epidemic, particularly long-term projections, are, with justification, viewed with a great deal of scepticism by most scientific authorities. Nevertheless, an analysis of the development of the epidemic until the present moment, coupled with a critical look at the biological properties of the virus as well as our present and also future options for treatment and vaccines, could all point to the unfurling of a biological holocaust of proportions similar to those of the classic plagues.

Epidemiological basis for a worst case scenario

As discussed on a number of previous occasions in this book, the ability of the virus to cause a progressive and permanent infection with permanent infectivity makes it a unique cause of epidemic disease. Thus, with no recovery, no loss of infectivity, no development of either individual or herd immunity, there is no known biological mechanism that can stop the continuing expansion of the disease unless an effective vaccine were to come about, and at present there is no feasible design for such an effective vaccine. The progressive increase in the pool of infectious virus can, in theory, only lead to an exponential increase in the number of individuals who will become infected until eventually the majority of the sexually active population will be infected unless interventions are at least moderately successful.

Disappointments in the available interventions

The major option for intervention which is available at present is education (Fig. 10.1). However, educational programmes and campaigns to effect behavioural changes to reduce the number of sexual partners, to practice safe sex and to promote usage of condoms have had mixed successes. A number of studies in communities and populations have demonstrated gratifying responses in reducing risk behaviour. This has been most striking among homosexual and bisexual men in San Francisco and also in a number of studies of similar populations in countries in the developed world. A few studies in Africa, for example of prostitutes in Nairobi, have also demonstrated positive responses, not least in the significantly increased usage of condoms as a result of educational programmes. More recently, however, studies have demonstrated a disconcerting return to high-risk behaviour, even in groups which had initially responded positively, such as the homosexual and bisexual men of San Francisco.

On the wider global scale, education has been largely unsuccessful in

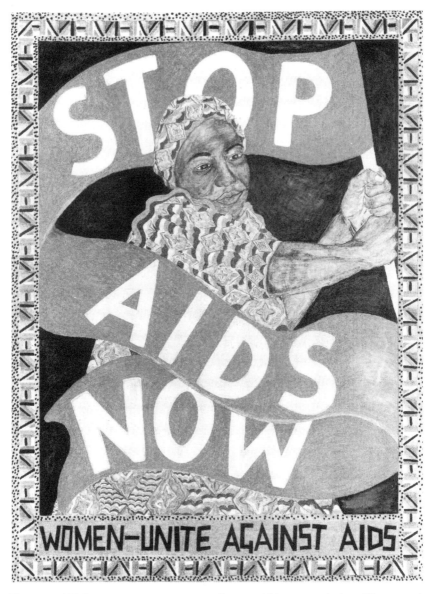

Fig. 10.1 AIDS awareness poster targeted to an African population. (Photograph courtesy of Johannesburg City AIDS Programme.)

effecting meaningful behaviour change, especially in the developing world. Of particular concern are the observations that although education has often achieved a greater awareness in African populations, it has failed to translate this into appropriate modifications in behaviour. To illustrate this, a study in rural Uganda found that even though 86% of the surveyed population understood the nature of sexual transmission of HIV, the HIV infection rate remained high.

Clearly, education on its own is insufficient to affect the transmission of HIV. Unfortunately much of what is needed to empower individuals to implement behaviour changes, of which there is often a high level of awareness, is absent, and socio-economic upliftment, improvements in housing especially for families of the providers of labour, and social programmes for women driven to prostitution (including alternative opportunities of earning income) are difficult enough in wealthy, developed nations, but are gargantuan tasks in poorer, developing countries. The enhancement of the status of women is similarly a particularly difficult problem in the male-dominated societies of the developing world where poverty and ignorance have entrenched age-old cultural prejudices.

Apparently insurmountable difficulties in drug and vaccine development

As discussed in Chapters 6 and 7, the biological properties of the virus, as well as its interaction with its host, impose unique difficulties for the development of curative drugs or preventative vaccines. Furthermore, even should a curative drug or effective vaccine become available, there is a despondency that the majority of developing countries would scarcely be in a financial position to derive significant benefit from any such breakthrough.

From the lessons of history it is difficult to conceptualize how the epidemic would be halted, let alone reversed, in the absence of a cheap curative drug or a cheap and effective preventative vaccine. The syphilis epidemic at the early part of the century displayed a similar kind of epidemiology to the present-day HIV epidemic. The campaigns which were initiated then closely paralleled those in place at present for HIV. For example, there were also vigorous educational programmes to reduce sexual high-risk behaviour, which were targeted at brothels and prostitutes as well as at military recruits to the United States Army. Scare tactics were commonly part and parcel of posters and pamphlets. Serological testing became obligatory before marriages could be licensed in certain states of the USA. All of these measures, however, had little appreciable effect on the expansion of the syphilis epidemic. It was only the advent of a cheap, safe and effective drug, penicillin, which eventually brought the epidemic under control.

Neglect of the Third World

By the end of this decade the WHO has predicted that over 90% of the worldwide burden of HIV will be shouldered by the developing world. Nevertheless, at present, fewer than 4% of scientific papers on HIV published in professional journals relate to the problems of AIDS in Africa. As the disparity between the load of AIDS on the health of nations widens even further between the developed world and the Third World, there is an increasing danger that the disease may, in the distant future, come to be considered even more as 'just another tropical disease' of the developing world. The attitudes between the developed and the developing countries of the world may come to parallel those seen at an individual level between the non-infected and the HIV-infected individual and a similar marginalization of developing countries could also eventuate.

A more realistic appraisal

The ceiling of infection

The WHO estimates that there are about a quarter to a half a billion heterosexuals who are at moderate to high risk of exposure to HIV because of multiple sexual partners. In addition, there are about ten million homosexuals and five million drug users who are also at moderate to high risk because of multiple sex partners or regular sharing of injection equipment.

At the other end of the risk scale, there is the segment of the population who have never had a sexually transmitted disease and who are at virtually no risk of acquiring one because of their sexual behaviour and habits, their avoidance of illicit drugs and the unlikelihood of their receiving unscreened blood. This segment of the population represents the uppermost ceiling of HIV infection into which the infection cannot penetrate. Thus, it is biologically impossible for the virus to affect anything approaching the entire population of a country, as a ceiling will always be present which will be a virtually impenetrable barrier to the spread of infection. Between these two poles of the high and almost no risk populations lies an intermediate level of population, who is at varying risk of contracting infection depending on the extent of the contact with the high-risk population and the extent of the pool of infection in the high-risk population. The future of the epidemic will therefore depend on the present and future size of each of these levels, the high-risk population, the intermediate population and the barrier, or ceiling, formed by the very low risk population.

The flattening of the epidemic curve

With the ageing of the epidemic, the natural consequences will be a progressive decrease in the number of non-infected individuals who fall into the high-risk groups, as those individuals who indulge in high-risk practices are likely to be the first to be infected, and most would already have been infected at a relatively early stage of the epidemic. The remnant of the population who are not infected will consist more and more of people at lower risks of infection. This will have the effect of progressively flattening the epidemic curve, which is a representation of the increase in the total number of cases.

The extent of contact between the intermediate zone and the high-risk zone will depend on the effectiveness of the educational efforts which aim to reduce high-risk behaviour. Similarly, the extent to which intermediate zone individuals will shift into the very low risk zone, and thereby expand the ceiling of infection, will also depend on the effectiveness of this education.

These population behavioural factors and their effects on the epidemiology of the virus are built into micro- and macro-simulation models, which compute the future progress of the infection. They were also used in the WHO Delphi projections for the future course of the epidemic. The WHO projections for the HIV epidemic in different parts of the world are characterized by epidemic curves which peak at different time points. Thus, in the homosexual population in developed countries, the peak took place in the latter half of the 1980s, and the rate of new infections has decreased significantly since then. In sub-Saharan Africa and in Latin America, the peak is optimistically expected in the late 1990s, while in Asia the peak may only occur early in the next century.

After the epidemic curve has peaked and the extent of new infections is on the wane, a baseline level will be reached where new non-infected individuals entering the high-risk zone will be vulnerable to infection and will then act as a reservoir of infection to contacts in the intermediate zone. The baseline level of continuing infection, as well as the risk of relapse of the epidemic, will depend on how well intervention programmes can be sustained.

Optimistic possibilities

The natural progress of the epidemic curve may well be drastically modified by future events which are presently not quantifiable.

Drug or vaccine breakthrough

The advent of a cheap, effective and safe drug or effective vaccine that could be put into widespread usage could drastically affect the progression of the epidemic.

A curative drug which would eliminate the infection from the body as well as being cheap and easily administered, such as penicillin is with syphilis, could, in theory, eliminate the infection. However, a drug which merely prevents the onset of AIDS or alleviates symptoms and does not reduce the excretion of the virus from the body may unwittingly even enhance the spread of infection. Because sexual transmission of HIV occurs predominantly in the stage of asymptomatic HIV infection and drops markedly when the individual becomes ill with AIDS, prolongation of this asymptomatic stage by a drug which does not eliminate the virus, or at least eliminate the virus from the sexual secretions and the bloodstream, could thus, in theory, contribute to the spread of the virus.

The effect of a vaccine on the overall epidemiology of HIV would also depend on whether the purpose of the vaccine is to protect against infection with HIV or to prevent individuals who are asymptomatically infected with HIV converting to AIDS. Vaccines that are cheap, safe and easy to administer as well as giving solid, long-lasting immunity against infection have had dramatic track records in controlling infectious diseases. They have totally eradicated one infectious disease – smallpox – and largely eliminated a number of others such as polio, diphtheria and, to a somewhat lesser extent, measles, mumps and rubella from the developed world and much of the developing world. An HIV vaccine with similar protective capabilities and logistics of administration could, in time, also have the same effect on the AIDS epidemic. In the short term there would, however, be little observable measure of success in terms of the number of AIDS cases over the following decade, until all those individuals who had already been infected with HIV before the advent of such a vaccine had converted to AIDS. The alternative vaccine approach, which utilizes vaccines to prevent individuals already infected with the virus from converting to AIDS, would have no effect on the overall epidemiology of the HIV epidemic and could, as in the case of a non-curative drug, theoretically enhance the spread of the virus, if it is not eliminated from sexual secretions or the bloodstream.

The most optimistic ideal to wish for would be the combination of an effective protective vaccine to interrupt the transmission of HIV in the human population and thereby curtail the epidemic of HIV infection, combined with a drug or another vaccine which would be used to prevent the conversion to AIDS in those individuals already infected. Theoretically, a protective vaccine could, as in the case of smallpox or as is possible within the next decade with poliomyelitis, totally eradicate the infection from the world. A curative drug, irrespective of how cheap, easy to administer, safe and effective it is, would be unable to eradicate the infection and thus the virus would always pose a threat of resurgence if it developed a resistance to the drug, or if control measures were to become lax. In the case of syphilis there has, in recent times, been such a resurgence, even though there has been no evidence of the organism having developed any resistance to penicillin.

The seemingly insurmountable hurdle of the costs of biological control of HIV, either by drugs or by vaccine, for the needs of the Third World is one where it is very difficult to conceptualize a solution, even in an optimistic scenario. To address this problem mankind would undoubtedly need to take a gigantic step forward, one which is perhaps even beyond the realms of present-day vision. Ultimately what would be needed is the transfer of vast sums of money and resources from the First to the Third World. In the future, AIDS may well become another challenge, as is protection of the environment, that has to be confronted by the developed world on behalf of the entire planet. The well-being of all will depend on the ability, the willingness and the adequacy of help which the First World will have to provide to the Third World, because infectious diseases, as with the earth's environment, are global issues. An optimistic scenario of AIDS control will therefore need to include not only a scientific breakthrough to develop a vaccine, but also a breakthrough in the global mindset of nations for a commitment to the single family of humankind.

Natural attenuation of HIV

There are two main factors which make an organism a successful parasite: one is efficient transmission, the other is the ability not to kill its host. Thus, a parasite which rapidly kills its host and is then not able to find another host will die off with its erstwhile host, whereas a parasite which keeps its host alive, and preferably healthy, will be in a better position to be transferred to as many other new susceptible individuals as possible if the host remains active and able to effectively spread the organism by its relevant transmission route. Thus, the natural tendency of organisms is to adapt to their host and to produce a progressively more attenuated (that is less severe) disease, the longer they have existed in that host species. This is borne out by many observations of infections in humans. For example, both smallpox and measles, as they moved from East to West, from ancient Rome to Europe and on to the New World, caused vast epidemics when newly introduced into susceptible populations and progressively decreased in their virulence as time passed. This adaptation to each population in turn would depend on how long in history the infectious organism had experience of that particular population. This is still clearly evident in diseases such as tuberculosis, which is well known to produce more severe disease in indigenous black Africans as compared to whites, and is probably related to the relatively recent introduction of the infection into Africa by Europeans who have built up a greater resistance because of many centuries of contact with the organism.

There is also some evidence that a natural attenuation process may operate similarly with HIV. SIV (simian immunodeficiency viruses) are all well adapted to their natural hosts, where they have presumably been present for long periods of time and do not cause disease. The only SIV strain which does cause disease is SIVmac, which is responsible for a lethal AIDS-like disease in Rhesus macaque monkeys. However, this virus has not been found in the wild macaque monkey in nature and the disease which is only seen in laboratory animals is probably an SIV strain from one of the other monkey species (possibly from the sooty mangebey monkey of West Africa, SIVsm). The disease in the macaque is therefore the result of the introduction of a virus into a new host species similar to that seen when infectious diseases are introduced into new human populations.

There is, not surprisingly, no evidence of any attenuation of HIV given its very recent history of infection in humankind. However, observations of the history of other human infectious diseases as well as the SIV do provide some basis for the optimism that the same tendencies could occur with HIV. One could, of course, also speculate on whether mutations could result in changes to the virus in the opposite direction, either that viruses could become more virulent or could learn the tricks of spread by other routes of transmission, such as breathing in air or ingesting food. Both of these nightmarish fears can be quite confidently allayed. As mentioned, the tendency of organisms is to mutate, for their own advantage, in the direction of greater attenuation rather than the reverse. If, theoretically, a virulent mutant were to arise which rapidly killed its host, it would be less likely to be transmitted to another host and, by a process of selection, would stand a greater chance of dying out. It is also highly improbable that HIV could affect the number of mutations which would be needed for it to change its biological features sufficiently to enable it to be transmitted successfully by other routes, such as via the respiratory or gastro-intestinal routes.

Conclusion

In the decade and a half that Man has been aware of this uniquely tragic disease, vastly different responses to it have been evident. Humankind as a whole has come to terms with the disease in a not dissimilar manner to the way in which an individual responds to HIV infection. Initially there is denial, an attempt to wish it away or underestimate its importance, or view it with a detachment of being a disease of 'others'. This is then followed by the phase of anger and a search for a scapegoat to apportion blame. Scapegoating, as discussed above, has characteristically been a response of humans to the plagues of history. Only after some experience of the epidemic over a sizeable period of time does the population mature into the acceptance phase. In this phase, opportunities to educate and change attitudes may be considerably better than at a later stage of resignation when 'burnout' and fatigue may well prevail.

With no other disease is research progress scrutinized so closely and reported so eagerly. Yet the true and significant progress in control will probably be concealed within the frequent cycles of anticipation and disappointment which follow the media reporting of 'breakthroughs'. It is certainly likely that the first preliminary results emanating from phase III vaccine trials may be prematurely and over-optimistically acclaimed only to be followed again by the familiar up and down cycle of 'breakthroughs' and disappointments. However, the immense increase in knowledge and the recent true breakthroughs in our fundamental understanding of the virus as well as the recent crucial demonstrations of the ability to overcome seemingly insurmountable obstacles to vaccine-induced protection gives much cause for optimism for the development of HIV vaccines reaching clinical trials by the end of the decade.

When the history of AIDS will come to be written some time in the future, the disease will undoubtedly be recorded as one of the greatest plagues of humankind. It will also have been tainted by the same fears, prejudices and bigotry that characterized the mediaeval plagues. Perhaps from the ashes of the AIDS epidemic may arise not only a vast knowledge of how to prevent and control persistent viral infections which attack the immune system, but also a new understanding and wisdom which will confirm to humankind that morality and expediency, pragmatism and justice, and utilitarianism and compassion are mutually beneficial goals, and also that disease and health bind all within the human family.

FURTHER READING

Introduction

Bygbjerg IC. AIDS in a Danish surgeon (Zaire, 1976). *Lancet* 1983; i: 925.

Desrosiers RC. HIV-I origins: a finger on the missing link. *Nature* 1990; **345**: 288–9.

Gallo RMD. *Virus hunting: Aids, cancer, and the human retrovirus: a story of scientific discovery*. Basic Books, 1993.

Garry RF, Witte MH, Gottlieb A *et al*. Documentation of an AIDS virus infection in the United States in 1968. *Journal of the American Medical Association* 1988; **260**: 2085–7.

Gosden RG. AIDS and malaria experiments. *Nature* 1992; **355**: 305.

Goudsmit J. *Viral sex: the nature of AIDS*. Oxford University Press, 1997.

Grmek MD. *History of AIDS: emergence and origin of a modern pandemic*. Princeton University Press, Princeton, New Jersey, 1990.

Koprowski H. My response to 'Polio vaccines and the origin of AIDS'. *Research in Virology* 1995; **146**: 233–4.

Levy JA, Pan L-Z, Beth-Giraldo E *et al*. Absence of antibodies to the human immuno-deficiency virus in sera from Africa prior to 1975. *Proceedings of the National Academy of Sciences* 1986; **83**: 7935–7.

Nahmias AJ, Weiss J, Yao X *et al*. Evidence for human infection with an HTLV III/LAV-like virus in Central Africa, 1959. *Lancet* 1986; ii: 1279–80.

Saxinger WC, Levine PH, Dean AG *et al*. Evidence for exposure to HTLV-III in Uganda before 1973. *Science* 1985; **227**: 1036–8.

Vandepitte J, Verwilghen R & Zachee P. AIDS and cryptococcosis (Zaire, 1977). *Lancet* 1983; i: 925–6.

Wain-Hobson S, Vartanian J-P, Henry M *et al*. LAV revisited: origins of the early HIV-1 isolates from Institut Pasteur. *Science* 1991; **252**: 961–5.

Zhu T & Ho DD. Was HIV present in 1959? *Nature* 1995; **374**: 503–4.

Chapter 1

Bartlett JG & Finkbeiner AK. *The guide to living with HIV infection: developed at the Johns Hopkins AIDS Clinic (Johns Hopkins Press Health Book)*. Johns Hopkins University Press, 1996.

Bowden F, Hoy J, Mijch A *et al. Fairfield Hospital HIV medicine handbook: a manual for clinicians working with HIV infection*. Melbourne University Press, 1995.

Centers for Disease Control and Prevention. 1994 revised classification system for human immunodeficiency virus infection in children less than 13 years of age. *Morbidity and Mortality Weekly Report* 1994; **43**: 1–11.

Centers for Disease Control and Prevention. 1997 USPHS/IDSA guidelines for the prevention of opportunistic infections in persons infected with human immunodeficiency virus. *Morbidity and Mortality Weekly Report* 1997; **46**: 1–46.

Devita VT Jr *et al.* (eds.) *AIDS: etiology, diagnosis, treatment and prevention*. Lippincott-Raven Publishers, 1996.

Greenspan D & Greenspan JS. HIV-related oral disease. *Lancet* 1996; **348**: 729–33.

Haas DW & Des Prez RM. Tuberculosis and acquired immunodeficiency syndrome: a historical perspective on recent developments. *The American Journal of Medicine* 1994; **96**: 439–50.

Kubler-Ross E. *AIDS: the ultimate challenge*. Collier Books, 1997.

Miller R. HIV-associated respiratory diseases. *Lancet* 1996; **348**: 307–12.

Price RW. Neurological complications of HIV infection. *Lancet* 1996; **348**: 445–52.

Sarraf D & Ernest JT. AIDS and the eyes. *Lancet* 1996; **348**: 525–8.

Schacker T, Collier AC, Hughes J *et al.* Clinical and epidemiologic features of primary HIV infection. *Annals of Internal Medicine* 1996; **125**: 257–64.

Schultz TF, Boshoff CH & Weiss RA. HIV infection and neoplasia. *Lancet* 1996; **348**: 587–91.

Sharpstone D & Gazzard B. Gastrointestinal manifestations of HIV infection. *Lancet* 1996; **348**: 379–83.

Sherr L (ed.). *Grief and AIDS*. John Wiley & Sons, 1995.

Stine GJ. *AIDS Update 1998: an annual overview of acquired immune deficiency syndrome (annual)*. Prentice Hall, 1998.

Tschachler E, Bergstresser PR & Stingl G. HIV-related skin diseases. *Lancet* 1996; **348**: 659–63.

World Health Organization. WHO case definitions for AIDS surveillance in adults and adolescents. *Weekly Epidemiological Record* 1994; **69**: 273–5.

Chapter 2

Barré-Sinoussi F. HIV as the cause of AIDS. *Lancet* 1996; **348**: 31–5.

Farrar GH, Roff MA, Amin T *et al.* Characterisation of a series of human immunodeficiency virus isolated derived sequentially from a single patient. *Journal of Medical Virology* 1991; **34**: 104–13.

Gelderblom HR. Assembly and morphology of HIV: potential effect of structure on viral function. *AIDS* 1991; **5**: 617–38.

Lever AML. HIV genetic variation: clinical importance. *Journal of Infection* 1997; **34**: 195–9.

Pepin J, Morgan G, Dunn D *et al.* HIV-1-induced immunosuppression among asymptomatic West African prostitutes: evidence that HIV-2 is pathogenic, but less so than HIV-1. *AIDS* 1991; **5**: 1165–72.

Pezo V & Wain-Hobson S. HIV genetic variation: life at the edge. *Journal of Infection* 1997; **34**: 201–3.

Smith DB, McAllister J, Casino C *et al.* Virus 'quasispecies': making a mountain out of a molehill? *Journal of General Virology* 1997; **78**: 1511–19.

Chapter 3

Cameron PU, Freudenthal PS, Barker JM *et al.* Dendritic cells exposed to human immuno-deficiency virus type-1 transmit a vigorous cytopathic infection to CD4+ T cells. *Science* 1992; **257**: 383–6.

Doms RW & Peipert SC. Unwelcomed guests with master keys: how HIV uses chemokine receptors for cellular entry. *Virology* 1997; **235**: 179–90.

Fauci AS. Host factors and the pathogenesis of HIV-induced disease. *Nature* 1996; **384**: 529–34.

Feinberg MB. Changing the natural history of HIV disease. *Lancet* 1996; **348**: 239–46.

Hanke T & Randall RE. Processing of viral proteins for presentation by molecules of the major histocompatibility complex. *Reviews in Medical Virology* 1994; **4**: 47–61.

Haynes BF, Pantaleo G, Fauci AS. Toward an understanding of the correlates of protective immunity to HIV infection. *Science* 1996; **271**: 324–8.

Meynard L, Otto SA, Jonker RR *et al.* Programmed death of T cells in HIV-1 infection. *Science* 1992; **257**: 217–19.

Moore JP. Coreceptors: implications for HIV pathogenesis and therapy. *Science* 1997; **276**: 51–2.

Oldstone MBA. How viruses escape from cytotoxic T lymphocytes: molecular parameters and players. *Virology* 1997; **234**: 179–85.

Oldstone MBA. HIV versus cytotoxic T lymphocytes – the war being lost. *The New England Journal of Medicine* 1997; **337**: 1306–8.

Schuitemaker H, Koot M, Kootstra NA *et al.* Biological phenotype of human immuno-deficiency virus type 1 clones at different stages of infection: progression of disease is associated with a shift from monocytotropic to T-cell-tropic virus populations. *Journal of Virology* 1992; **66**: 1354–60.

Chapter 4

Barnett T & Blaikie P. *AIDS in Africa: its present and future impact.* Belhaven, 1992.

Centers for Disease Control Recommendations for preventing transmission of human immuno-deficiency virus and hepatitis B virus to patients during exposure-prone invasive procedures. *Morbidity and Mortality Weekly Report* 1991; **40**: 1–9.

Coyle SL *et al.* (eds.) *Evaluating AIDS: prevention programs.* National Academy Press, Washington, 1991.

Dunn DT, Newell ML, Ades AE *et al.* Risk of human immunodeficiency virus type 1 transmission through breastfeeding. *Lancet* 1992; **340**: 585–8.

Ekstrand ML. Safer sex maintenance among gay men: are we making any progress? *AIDS* 1990; **4**: 645–50.

Gershon RRM, Vlahov D & Nelson KE. The risk of transmission of HIV-1 through non-percutaneous, non-sexual modes – a review. *AIDS* 1990; **4**: 645–50.

John GC & Kreiss J. Mother-to-child transmission of human immunodeficiency virus type 1. *Epidemiologic Reviews* 1996; **18**: 149–57.

Laga M, Alary M, Nzila N *et al.* Condom promotion, sexually transmitted diseases treatment, and declining incidence of HIV-1 infection in female Zairian sex workers. *Lancet* 1994; **344**: 246–8.

Mastro TD & de Vincenzi I. Probabilities of sexual HIV-1 transmission. *AIDS* 1996; 10: S75–S82.

O'Shea S, Rostron T, Mullen JE *et al.* Stability of infectious HIV in clinical samples and isolation from small volumes of whole blood. *Journal of Clinical Pathology* 1994; **47**: 152–4.

Plummer FA, Simonsen JN, Cameron DW *et al.* Cofactors in male-female sexual transmission of human immunodeficiency virus type 1. *Journal of Infectious Diseases* 1991; **163**: 233–9.

Royce RA, Sena A, Cates W *et al.* Sexual transmission of HIV. *New England Journal of Medicine* 1997; **336**: 1072–8.

Scarlatti G. Paediatric HIV infection. *Lancet* 1996; **348**: 863–8.

Schreiber GB, Busch MP, Kleinman SH *et al.* The risk of transfusion-transmitted viral infections. *New England Journal of Medicine* 1996; **334**: 1686–90.

Sepkowitz KA. Occupationally acquired infections in health care workers. Part I. *Annals of Internal Medicine* 1996; **125**: 826–34.

Sepkowitz KA. Occupationally acquired infections in health care workers. Part II. *Annals of Internal Medicine* 1996; **125**: 917–28.

Sperling RS, Shapiro DE, Coombs RW *et al.* Maternal viral load, zidovudine treatment, and the risk of transmission of human immunodeficiency virus type 1 from mother to infant. *New England Journal of Medicine* 1996; **335**: 1621–9.

van Bueren J, Simpson RA, Jacobs P *et al.* Survival of human immunodeficiency virus in suspension and dried onto surfaces. *Journal of Clinical Microbiology* 1994; **32**: 571–4.

Voeller B, Nelson J, Day C. Viral leakage risk differences in latex condoms. *AIDS Research and Human Retroviruses* 1994; **10**: 701–10.

Webb PA, Happ CM, Maupin GO *et al.* Potential for insect transmission of HIV: experimental exposure of *Cimex hemipterus* and *Toxorhynchites amboinensis* to human immunodeficiency virus. *Journal of Infectious Diseases* 1989; **160**: 970–7.

Chapter 5

Bloom DE & Glied S. Benefits and costs of HIV testing. *Science* 1991; **252**: 1798–804.

Centers for Disease Control. Interpretation and use of the Western blot assay for sero-diagnosis of human immunodeficiency virus type 1 infections. *Morbidity and Mortality Weekly Report* 1989; **38**: 1–7.

Centers for Disease Control and Prevention. 1997 revised guidelines for performing CD4+ T-cell determinations in persons infected with human immunodeficiency virus (HIV). *Morbidity and Mortality Weekly Report* 1997; **46**: 1.

Gürtler L. Difficulties and strategies of HIV diagnosis. *Lancet* 1996; **348**: 176–9.

Gwinn M, Redus MA, Granade TC *et al.* HIV-1 serologic test results for one million newborn dried-bloodspecimens: assay performance and implications for screening. *Journal of Acquired Immune Deficiency Syndromes* 1992; **5**: 505–11.

Hammer S, Crumpacker C, D'Aquila R *et al.* Use of virologic assays for detection of human immunodeficiency virus in clinical trials: recommendations of the AIDS Clinical Trials Group virology committee. *Journal of Clinical Microbiology*; 1993; **31**: 2557–64.

Mellors JW, Rinaldo CR, Gupta P *et al.* Prognosis in HIV-1 infection predicted by the quantity of virus in plasma. *Science* 1996; **272**: 1167–70.

Merson MH, Feldman EA, Bayer R *et al.* Rapid self testing for HIV infection. *Lancet* 1996: **348**: 352–3.

Morens D. Editorial response: serological screening tests for antibody to human immunodeficiency virus – the search for perfection in an imperfect world. *Clinical Infectious Diseases* 1997; **25**: 101–3.

Mortimer PP & Parry JV. Detection of antibody to HIV in saliva: a brief review. *Clinical and Diagnostic Virology* 1994; **2**: 231–43.

Owens DK, Holodniy M, Garber AM *et al.* Polymerase chain reaction for the diagnosis of HIV infection in adults: a meta-analysis with recommendations for clinical practice and study design. *Annals of Internal Medicine* 1996; **124**: 803–15.

Saag MS. Use of virologic markers in clinical practice. *Journal of Acquired Immune Deficiency Syndromes and Human Retrovirology* 1997; **16**: S3–S13.

Schochetman G, George JR (eds.). *AIDS testing: a comprehensive guide to technical, medical, social, legal, and management issues.* Springer Verlag, 1994.

Tribble DR, Rodier GR, Saad MD *et al.* Comparative field evaluation of HIV rapid diagnostic assays using serum, urine, and oral mucosal transudate specimens. *Clinical and Diagnostic Virology* 1997; **7**: 127–32.

World Health Organization. Joint United Nations Programme on HIV/AIDS (UNAIDS) – WHO. *Weekly Epidemiological Record* 1997; **72**: 81–8.

Chapter 6

Abrams DI. Alternative therapies in HIV infection. *AIDS* 1990; **4**: 1179–87.

Brandt AM. The syphilis epidemic and its relation to AIDS. *Science* 1988; **239**: 375–80.

Carpenter CCJ, Fischi MA, Hammer SM *et al.* Antiretroviral therapy for HIV infection in 1997. *Journal of the American Medical Association* 1997; **277**: 1962–9.

Centers for Disease Control and Prevention. Recommendations of the U.S. Public Health Service task force on the use of zidovudine to reduce perinatal transmission of human immunodeficiency virus. *Morbidity and Mortality Weekly Report* 1994; **43**: 1–20.

Centers for Disease Control and Prevention. Case-control study of HIV seroconversion in health-care workers after percutaneous exposure to HIV-infected blood – France, United Kingdom, and United States, January 1988 – August 1994. *Morbidity and Mortality Weekly Report* 1995; **44**: 929–36.

Centers for Disease Control and Prevention. Update: provisional public health service recommendations for chemoprophylaxis after occupational exposure to HIV. *Morbidity and Mortality Weekly Report* 1996; **45**: 468–72.

Cohn JA. Recent advances in HIV infection – I. *British Medical Journal* 1997; **314**: 487–91.

Deeks SG, Smith M, Holodniy M *et al.* HIV-1 protease inhibitors. A review for clinicians. *Journal of the American Medical Association* 1997; **277**: 145–53.

Gazzard BG, Moyle GJ, Johnson M *et al.* British HIV Association guidelines for antiretro-viral treatment of HIV seropositive individuals. *Lancet* 1977; **349**: 1086–92.

Gerberding JL. Prophylaxis for occupational exposure to HIV. *Annals of Internal Medicine* 1996; **125**: 497–501.

Lipsky JJ. Antiretroviral drugs for AIDS. *Lancet* 1996; **348**: 800–3.

Steinbrook R. Battling HIV on many fronts. *New England Journal of Medicine* 1997; **337**: 779–81.

Wurtman RJ. What went right: why is HIV a treatable infection? *Nature Medicine* 1997; **3**: 714–7.

Chapter 7

Anderson RM & Garnett GP. Low-efficacy HIV vaccines: potential for community-based intervention programmes. *Lancet* 1996; **348**: 1010–13.

Bangham CRM & Phillips RE. What is required of an HIV vaccine? *Lancet* 1997; **350**: 1617–21.

Bloom BR. The highest attainable standard: ethical issues in AIDS vaccines. *Science* 1998; **279**: 186–8.

Cranage MP, Baskerville A, Ashworth LAE *et al.* Intrarectal challenge of macaques vaccinated with formalin-inactivated simian immunodeficiency virus. *Lancet* 1992; **339**: 273–4.

Esparza J, Heyward WL, Osmanov S. HIV vaccine development: from basic research to human trials. *AIDS* 1996; **10**: S123–S32.

Girard M, Kieny M-P, Pinter A *et al.* Immunization of chimpanzees confers protection against challenge with human immunodeficiency virus. *Proceedings of the National Academy of Sciences* 1991; **88**: 542–6.

Haynes BF. HIV vaccines: where we are and where we are going. *Lancet* 1996; **348**: 933–7.

Heeney JL. Primate models for AIDS vaccine development. *AIDS* 1996; **10**: S115–S22.

Johnston MI. HIV/AIDS vaccine development: challenges, progress and future directions. *Reviews in Medical Virology* 1996; **6**: 123–140.

Lambert P-H & Siegrist C-A. Vaccines and vaccination. *British Medical Journal* 1997; **315**: 1595–8.

Robinson HL. Nucleic acid vaccines: an overview. *Vaccine* 1997; **15**: 785–7.

Chapter 8

Bayer R. As the second decade of AIDS begins: an international perspective on the ethics of the epidemic. *AIDS* 1992; **6**: 527–32.

Bayer R & Healton C. Controlling AIDS in Cuba: the logic of quarantine. *New England Journal of Medicine* 1989; **320**: 1022–4.

Burris S, Dalton HL, Miller JL (eds.) *AIDS law today: a new guide for the public.* Yale University Press, 1993.

Centers for Disease Control and Prevention. U.S. Public Health Service recommendations for human immunodeficiency virus counselling and voluntary testing for pregnant women. *Morbidity and Mortality Weekly Report* 1995; **44**: 1–15.

Dancaster JT & Dancaster LA. Confidentiality concerning HIV/AIDS status – the implications of the Appeal Court decision. *South African Medical Journal* 1995; **85**: 141–4.

Gostin LO, Lazzarini Z, Gostin Lawrence O. *Human rights and public health in the AIDS pandemic.* Oxford University Press, 1997.

Jayasuriya DC. Worldwide review of restrictions placed upon people with HIV/AIDS. *Reviews in Medical Virology* 1992; **2**: 191–4.

Shilts R. *And the band played on: politics, people, and the AIDS epidemic.* Penguin USA, 1995.

Temmerman M, Ndinya-Achola J, Ambani J *et al.* The right not to know HIV-test results. *Lancet* 1995; **345**: 969–70.

Wachter RM. AIDS, activism, and the politics of health. *New England Journal of Medicine* 1992; **326**: 128–33.

Zion D. Ethical considerations of clinical trials to prevent vertical transmission of HIV in developing countries. *Nature Medicine* 1998; **4**: 11–12.

Chapter 9

Anderson R. AIDS: trends, predictions, controversy. *Nature* 1993; **363**: 393–4.

Buehler JW, Berkelman RL & Stehr-Green JK. The completeness of AIDS surveillance. *Journal of Acquired Immune Deficiency Syndromes* 1992; **5**: 257–64.

Chin J, Sato PA & Mann JM. Projections of HIV infections and AIDS cases to the year 2000. *Bulletin of the World Health Organization* 1990; **68**: 1–11.

Gertig DM, Marion SA & Schechter MT. Estimating the extent of under-reporting in AIDS surveillance. *AIDS* 1991; **5**: 1157–64.

Gupta S & Anderson R. Sex, AIDS and mathematics. *New Scientist* 1992; **135**: 34–8.

Hendriks JCM, Medley GF, Heisterkamp SH *et al.* Short-term predictions of HIV prevalence and AIDS incidence. *Epidemiology and Infection* 1992; **109**: 149–60.

Karon JM, Rosenberg PS, McQuillan G *et al.* Prevalence of HIV infection in the United States, 1984 to 1992. *Journal of the American Medical Association* 1996; **276**: 126–31.

Mann J & Tarantola DJM (eds.) *AIDS in the World II: global dimensions, social roots, and responses: the global AIDS policy coalition.* Oxford University Press, 1996.

Mertens TE & Burton A. Estimates and trends of the HIV/AIDS epidemic. *AIDS* 1996; **10**: S221–8.

Mertens TE & Low-Beer D. HIV and AIDS: where is the epidemic going? *Bulletin of the World Health Organization* 1996; **74**: 121–9.

Quinn TC. Global burden of the HIV pandemic. *Lancet* 1996; **348:** 99–106.

Weniger BG & Brown T. The march of AIDS through Asia. *New England Journal of Medicine* 1996; **335:** 343–4.

World Health Organization. Global AIDS surveillance Part I. *Weekly Epidemiological Record* 1997; **72:** 357–64.

World Health Organization. Global AIDS surveillance Part II. *Weekly Epidemiological Record* 1997; **72:** 365–72.

Wortley PM & Fleming PL. AIDS in women in the United States. *Journal of the American Medical Association* 1997; **278:** 911–6.

Chapter 10

Bayer R. Public health policy and the AIDS epidemic. *New England Journal of Medicine* 1991; **324:** 1500–4.

Coates TJ, Aggleton P, Gutzwiller F *et al*. HIV prevention in developed countries. *Lancet* 1996; **348:** 1143–8.

d'Cruz-Grote D. Prevention of HIV infection in developing countries. *Lancet* 1996; **348:** 1071–4.

Editorial. AIDS: the third wave. *Lancet* 1994; **343:** 186–8.

Editorial. HIV: a war still to be won. *Lancet* 1996; **348:** 1.

Hearst N & Mandel JS. A research agenda for AIDS prevention in the developing world. *AIDS* 1997; **11:** S1–S4.

Hurley SF, Kaldor JM, Gardiner S *et al*. Lifetime cost of human immunodeficiency virus-related health care. *Journal of Acquired Immune Deficiency Syndromes and Human Retrovirology* 1996; **12:** 371–8.

Nelson KE, Celentano DD, Eiumtrakol S *et al*. Changes in sexual behaviour and a decline in HIV infection among young men in Thailand. *New England Journal of Medicine* 1996; **335:** 297–303.

INDEX

active surveillance 154, 224–5, 228–9
acute cytocidal infections 54
acute HIV syndrome 33–4, 88
  CNS manifestations 37
acyclovir 159, 160, 161
adenovirus 191
Africa, AIDS origins 13–14
African AIDS 22–4
African swine fever virus (ASFV) 6
AIDS 35, 246–8
  classification systems 36–7, 41
  discovery of causal agent 4–9
  fearsome characteristics of 18–19
  history of 1–4
  origins of 12–18
  public health laws and 206–9
  see also epidemiology; HIV
AIDS dementia 39, 40, 86
AIDS tests 126–56
  benefits of 156
  bloodbank screening 152–3
  diagnostic testing in practice 151–2
  false-positive test results 127–8, 147
  history of 127–30
  immunological function evaluation
    148–51
  lymphocyte enumeration 149–59
  lymphocyte functional analysis 150
  surrogate markers 150–1
  in infants 154–5
  patient monitoring 155
  serological techniques 82, 132–7,
    139–40
  laboratory diagnosis of HIV infection
    143–8
  sensitivity and specificity of 138

see also ELISA (enzyme-linked
    immunosorbent assay)
  surveillance and 153–4
  viral detection techniques 130–2
  laboratory diagnosis of HIV infection
    138–43
  viral load tests 140, 142–3
  see also screening programmes
AIDS virus see HIV (human
    immunodeficiency virus)
AIDS-related complex (ARC) 33, 35
AL 721 176
amantadine 160, 162
amniocentesis 120
ampligen 165, 176
amyl nitrite 4
animal models 196–9
  chimpanzee model 196–7
  macaque model 197–9
anti-sense nucleotides 172–3
antibacterial agents 158–9
antibodies 79, 81, 89
  see also immunoglobulins
antibody enhancement 193
antibody titre 133
antibody-dependent cytotoxic cells (ADCC)
    79
antigen detection tests 132–7, 139–40
  see also ELISA (enzyme-linked
    immunosorbent assay)
antigen-presenting cells 76, 79–80, 83,
    188
antimicrobial drugs, theoretical basis of
    157–8
  see also antiretroviral therapy; antiviral
    drug development

266